Obesity

Life Beyond the GLP-1 Injection

Dr. Tom Barber
University Hospitals Coventry and Warwickshire NHS Trust and University of Warwick
Coventry, UK

WILEY

This edition first published 2027

Registered Offices
John Wiley & Sons, Inc., 111 River Street, Hoboken, NJ 07030, USA
John Wiley & Sons Ltd, New Era House, 8 Oldlands Way, Bognor Regis, West Sussex, PO22 9NQ, UK

For details of our global editorial offices, customer services, and more information about Wiley products visit us at www.wiley.com.

The manufacturer's authorized representative according to the EU General Product Safety Regulation is Wiley-VCH GmbH, Boschstr. 12, 69469 Weinheim, Germany, e-mail: Product_Safety@wiley.com.

Wiley also publishes its books in a variety of electronic formats and by print-on-demand. Some content that appears in standard print versions of this book may not be available in other formats.

Library of Congress Cataloging-in-Publication Data Applied for

Paperback ISBN: 9781394391042

Cover Design: Wiley
Cover Image: Sara S. Watson

Set in 11.5/13.5pt STIXTwoText by Straive, Pondicherry, India

Printed and bound by CPI Group (UK) Ltd, Croydon, CR0 4YY

C9781394391042_250926

Contents

About the Author and Illustrator

Author

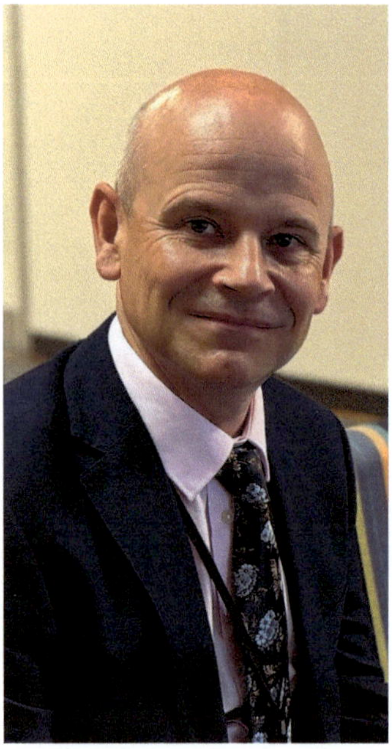

Dr. Tom Barber qualified as a medical doctor in 1998, with an MA (Hons) in Medical Sciences from *Cambridge University* (Christ's College) and MBBS in Clinical Medicine from *Newcastle University*. He was awarded a DPhil (on the topic of Polycystic Ovary Syndrome) from the *University of Oxford* (St. Edmund Hall) in 2007. Dr Barber leads the tier 3 obesity service at *University Hospitals Coventry and Warwickshire NHS Trust*, a major academic teaching hospital in the United Kingdom (since 2010) and has worked as a medical doctor in the UK-based NHS setting for over 27 years. As a Consultant Endocrinologist, he has managed many thousands of people living with obesity, obesity-related conditions like Type 2 Diabetes and other endocrine (hormonal) problems. In 2024, Dr Barber was awarded a *National (N2) Clinical Impact Award* (the second highest level in the UK), reflecting excellence in clinical delivery, innovation, research, teaching and impact. Dr Barber is a Professor of Endocrinology (affiliated with *University of Warwick* and *Coventry University*), *Fellow of the Royal College of Physicians* (London), *Fellow of the Association of Physicians of Great Britain and Ireland,* and *Fellow of the Higher Education Academy*. Dr Barber has published >170 scientific papers in leading peer-reviewed journals in the field of obesity, diabetes and metabolism with >11,700 citations, and in 2025 was recognised by '*ScholarGPS*' as a globally highly ranked scholar in the field of obesity (based on scientific publications and citations), placing him in the top 0.05% of scholars. Dr Barber is Editor-in-Chief for a peer-reviewed journal (*Expert Review in Endocrinology and Metabolism*) and regularly leads a teaching block on obesity for medical students at *Warwick Medical School.* Dr Barber engages frequently with national and other media outlets on obesity-related topics, including numerous podcasts, commissioned articles and appearances on all the major terrestrial TV channels in the United Kingdom.

Illustrator

Sara Watson is a first-time illustrator currently studying Art History at the *University of St Andrews*. Her work reflects an interest in cross-disciplinary approaches to visual storytelling, influenced by her studies in Art, Biology and English Literature at A level. She has a long-standing interest in art and visual culture and was awarded the Drawing Prize in her final year at school. Through illustration, Sara enjoys exploring ways of bringing multifaceted ideas to life and is particularly interested in visual communication across the arts as she continues to develop her creative expression.

Preface

Information is instantly available to us, and everyone has a platform irrespective of their credentials. The result is lots of misinformation. In the case of obesity, there are lots of fad diets and fake promises out there, and we are like rabbits startled in the headlights, not knowing which way to turn. In recent times, obesity has become an important issue in our society, with much media attention fuelled by the rise of the GLP-1 injections ('skinny jabs'). This, combined with the misinformation and many misconceptions about obesity in our society, formed a key rationale for me to write this book. Written for everyone, and by a true expert in obesity with nearly three decades of experience of managing many thousands of people living with obesity, this book provides clear and helpful advice for anyone interested in obesity and its effective management. Each chapter addresses an important topic, including everything you need to know about the GLP-1 injections ('skinny jabs'), the thorny and misunderstood topic of diet, physical exercise, fibre and how to look after your muscles. As a doctor, my job involves a holistic approach (relating to the whole person). Rather than just focusing on one specific area, this book also adopts a holistic approach to obesity management, by joining together all the individual jigsaw pieces. The complete picture can then be understood and used as a guide by all. Join me on a journey that lifts us out of the startling headlights and into the driving seat, with a clear and unobstructed view of the road ahead.

Dr. Tom Barber
Coventry, England
March 2026

Acknowledgements

I have wanted to write a book on obesity for many years. Luckily for me, and for all my readers, this opportunity presented itself with a 'star alignment' in early 2025. I have so many people to thank for this and will do my best to include them all here.

Firstly, I would like to thank my patients who have provided much of the inspiration for me to write this book. I would also like to thank my excellent colleagues based at *University Hospitals Coventry and Warwickshire NHS Trust*, United Kingdom. This includes my colleagues within the wider obesity multidisciplinary team and those based at the *Warwickshire Institute for the Study of Diabetes, Endocrinology and Metabolism* (*WISDEM*) centre. I would also like to thank the 'Communications' team at the *University of Warwick* and Professor Simon Barnes (*Warwick Business School, University of Warwick*) for their initial guidance and support in the early stages of securing a willing publisher.

Next, I would like to thank my publisher *Wiley*, including the editorial team for their agreement to publish this book, and the entire production team for their excellent input. Specifically, I would like to thank Emily Tapp (Commissioning Editor), Calee Sears (Editorial Assistant), Harini Arumugam (Managing Editor), and Jamila Niroop (Content Refinement Specialist) for their ongoing and invaluable help, support and guidance in the production of this book.

Any book needs figures and illustrations. For this, I have been blessed and incredibly fortunate to have Sara Watson who has prepared most of the figures in this book. Sara's artistic prowess, creativity and skill have surpassed all expectations and have brought this book to life. Sara, thank you so much. You have a great future ahead of you!

Finally, I want to thank my family and loved ones, of whom I am grateful and incredibly proud, and love each one. Simon and Robin, for providing their honest opinions of early drafts of chapters in a way that only brothers can do. My two boys, Harry and Joshua, for their support and encouragement. My parents, Susan and George, for providing opinions and suggestions on early drafts. Freya, Zara and Sofia for their support and encouragement, and my partner, Liz, who has supported and encouraged me throughout, including opinions and suggestions on early drafts. Thank you, Liz! Finally, thank you to Ziggy, our Miniature Poodle, who has provided so many people with unwavering love, joy and loyalty. Thank you, Ziggy! We can all learn from you.

I would also like to thank you, dear reader. Our modern-day world seems increasingly divided and fractured. With this in mind, we can all strive and aspire to be the change we want to see.

Forgive without limits;
Love without condition.

1 Obesity: A Global Health Problem

The global obesity problem and I are the same age. I was born in the early 1970s, and back then global obesity wasn't really a problem. There have always existed people living with obesity, including extreme forms of obesity, even in antiquity. This is evidenced by the 'Venus' figurines depicting obesity from the Upper Paleolithic period, tens of thousands of years ago (*fig 1.1*). Unlike in our modern-day environment, back then obesity was probably viewed as a sign of fertility, survival and resilience in the context of climate change, nutritional stress and starvation. For much of our evolution though, obesity would have been uncommon and unusual. Today in the United Kingdom at the time of writing, obesity now affects one in four adults, global prevalence of obesity exceeds 890 million and overweight affects 2.5 billion adults (1). In just 50 years, the prevalence of global obesity within our species has gone from being uncommon to common. Indeed, obesity is now the most important health crisis of our time and is classified as a non-infectious global pandemic by the World Health Organisation (WHO) (2). Obesity contributes towards the development of >50 obesity-related conditions (most notably Type 2 Diabetes Mellitus [T2D]) and multiple malignancies (3, 4). Obesity confers a substantial health economic burden (5), diminishes work productivity (6), psychosocial functioning (7) and overall well-being and quality of life.

This book is written for anyone who wants to truly understand obesity, and by implication what has happened to our species since the early 1970s, and the future prevention and management of obesity. Whilst useful for healthcare professionals and students involved in the management of people living with obesity, I have written this book for everyone. My aim throughout is to improve the public understanding of obesity and to dispel commonly held misconceptions. And so many misconceptions! Alas, some of these misconceptions may even be held and spread by healthcare professionals themselves, who are not immune. It is interesting to speculate where these misconceptions may have come from. Ultimately, ignorance plays an important role, of course. On that note, I do not profess to have all the answers, and indeed there are aspects of obesity that remain incompletely understood. When faced

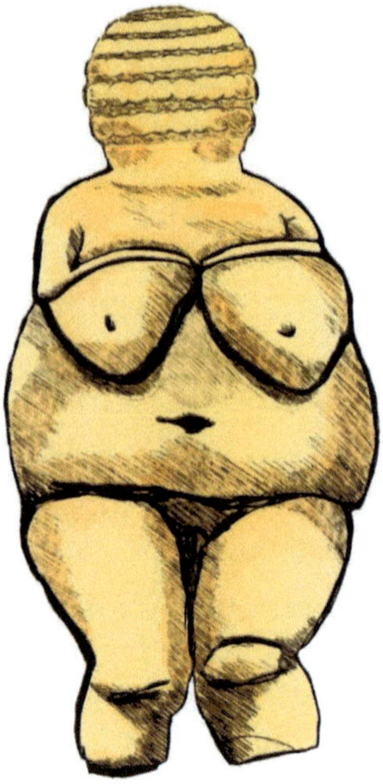

Figure 1.1: Venus of Willendorf.

with such unknowns though, we should acknowledge them rather than making up an incorrect story or conspiracy to fill any gaps in our knowledge, however tempting or comforting this latter approach may be. Then there is social media, with its emphasis on voice and opinion, in which everyone can be an 'expert'. This can turbocharge the spread and promulgation of misinformation and misconceptions.

Obesity is complex. There are multiple components. In this book, I have chosen each chapter to cover key aspects of obesity. In Chapter 2, I discuss how our appetite is regulated, why appetite is central to our body weight, why many of us struggle to maintain our body weight following weight loss and why appetite is not really something that we can easily control consciously, contrary to common belief. In Chapter 3, I discuss Body Mass Index (BMI) as a key measure that is used throughout the world to define obesity and to prioritise treatment strategies for obesity. I will discuss how BMI is a flawed measure for the individual and argue for a transformation in the way in which we define obesity and prioritise therapies, through future measures that reflect overall body composition and cardiovascular risk. In Chapter 4, I discuss the important role of our skeletal muscles in metabolic health and how they have become forgotten in obesity management, eclipsed by our focus on fat tissue and its diminution. I will discuss how we can optimise our skeletal muscle mass as we get older, to help in obesity prevention, management and overall health and well-being. In Chapter 5, I discuss the strange and hidden gut microbiota and how this influences our health and well-being, including our appetite and metabolic regulation, and the importance of establishing and maintaining a healthy gut microbiota. In Chapter 6, I discuss how our sleep affects our appetite and how getting a good night's sleep should be the first step to obesity management. I argue that the common (and rather unhelpful and irritating) mantra 'eat less, do more' should be prefixed (and maybe even replaced) by 'sleep more'. In Chapter 7, I discuss physical exercise and its role in obesity management and appetite control. In Chapter 8, I discuss the importance of dietary fibre not just for our gut health, but for all aspects of our health, and how in the western world we have become fibre impoverished and how we can address this important nutritional deficiency in the future. In Chapter 9, I discuss the art of listening in all its forms and argue that in our modern-day stressful and chaotic environments with all its distractions, we have lost our ability to listen. I discuss the importance of re-learning this key life skill for our health, well-being and body weight and composition. In Chapter 10, I discuss the rise of drug therapies for obesity (GLP-1 injections or 'skinny jabs'), with all its unprecedented media attention. I discuss the mechanisms of action of these therapies, their efficacy, safety and tolerability, and the future of pharmacotherapies for obesity, including some of the novel molecules in development. In Chapter 11, I discuss the thorny and challenging topic of diet and provide advice based on our best scientific evidence. Finally, in Chapter 12, I discuss the importance of our environment for our body weight and illustrate a future 'leptogenic' environment that would address the current global obesity problem and help to prevent weight gain and obesity in future generations.

All that to come. There is a lot to get through. In the remainder of this opening chapter though, I will discuss three key aspects of obesity. The first relates to the definition of obesity: what is it? The second relates to the origin of obesity: what has caused the global obesity problem? This discussion will impel us to consider commonly held misconceptions of obesity as a 'lifestyle choice' and then to discuss the third aspect: the stigmatisation of obesity.

The Definition of Obesity: What Is It?

How do you define an elephant? This question is harder to answer than it seems. You might say that it is a large mammal with a trunk and tusks. But these would be merely descriptive terms, and not useful from a defining perspective. The problem is that other animals may have some similar elephant-like features, like the extinct woolly mammoth for example, and this would diminish their defining qualities (*fig 1.2*). You may devise some scale of elephantness, with a sophisticated algorithm where you can input data on features like trunk and tusk size, speed of walking, hairiness,

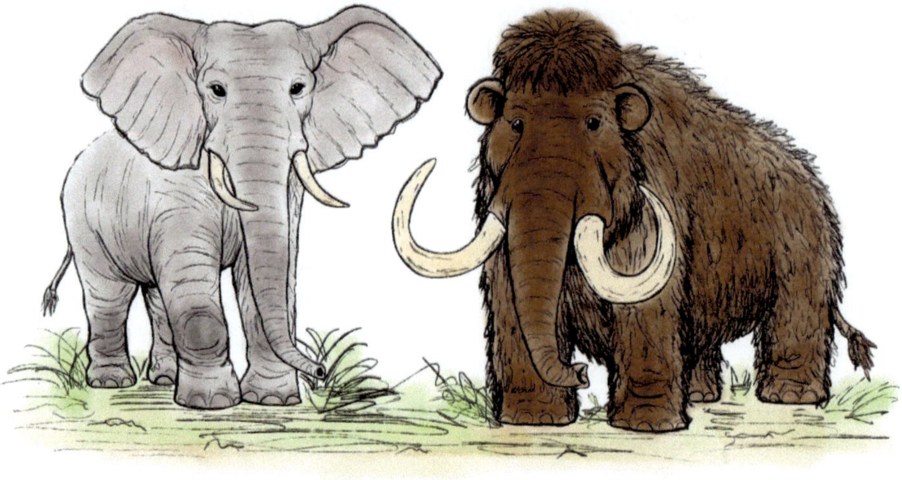

Figure 1.2: Elephant versus Woolly Mammoth. Elephants and woolly mammoths each have similarities like presence of tusks and a trunk and four legs. However, there are distinct differences including size of ears, hairiness and the size and shape of the tusks. As humans, we don't need sophisticated algorithms to tell the difference between an elephant and a woolly mammoth. We can see these instantly and recognise each as different mammals.

ear size and body weight, for example, and it would then churn out a probability that the thing you are looking at is indeed an elephant (rather than a woolly mammoth or some other elephant-like mammal). But this would just be another sophisticated way of using descriptors for definition. To properly define an elephant, you would probably need to go down to the DNA level. (In fact, it is through DNA analysis that new species are identified nowadays, and how we can gain insights into our evolutionary history and the relatedness between species. This technique has thrown up some surprises including that whales and hippopotamuses are each other's closest living relatives). In reality of course, we do not need to resort to such DNA-based techniques. Of all our flaws and susceptibilities to aberrant mental processing and misconceptions, our species is particularly adept at visual pattern recognition, and by implication the correct identification of and discernment between elephants, woolly mammoths and other objects in our visual world. We can look at an elephant and know immediately that it is an elephant without taking out a tape measure or resorting to any fancy algorithm. We are so adept at this task, in fact, that we often take for granted this almost 'superhuman' ability. One of the key challenges for engineers who work on developing the driverless cars of the future is to teach the cars' 'visual' systems how to identify and recognise correctly objects within their immediate environment including a pedestrian who suddenly walks out in front of the car.

In a similar way to identifying elephants and other objects through our vision, most of us are pretty good at visually recognising a person living with obesity. However, to move a step beyond that initial visual recognition and drill down into how we define obesity, we come up with the same problems we identified with the elephant example outlined earlier. We may use descriptive terms like the shape and size of the abdomen, for example, or the girth of the limbs, or size of the neck and face, but these are just descriptors and don't really help with definition.

Some conditions in medicine are relatively easy to define. Perhaps the simplest are those 'monogenic' conditions, in which a mutation or variant in a single gene results in a particular condition. There are many examples of such monogenic conditions, including within my own specialty of endocrinology. One example is 'Autosomal Dominant Hypocalcaemia' in which the calcium-sensing receptor does not work correctly, and this can lead to problems with abnormal calcium levels in the blood. Although descriptive terms can be used for these conditions, diagnostically we can simply look at the gene in question and determine whether there is a mutation. In this way, we can use monogenic gene mutations to both diagnose and define certain conditions. The problem with obesity, and for many other conditions in medicine for that matter, is that its underlying pathogenesis (the mechanisms by which a disease becomes clinically manifest) is complex and does not rely simply on a single-gene mutation. At least not for most people living with obesity. (In fact, there are some rare monogenic forms of obesity in which definition is much easier, based on the presence of a single-gene mutation (8)).

A monogenic gene mutation is an example of a discrete variable. Either you have it, or you don't. A bit like an 'on/off' switch. This makes definition relatively easy. However, much of biology and pathology does not work like this. Indeed, any pathological or biological attribute that has multiple and complex underlying causal factors tends to manifest clinically more like a 'dimmer switch' than an 'on/off' switch. We call this a 'continuous variable'. An example would be height within any population. Adult height is influenced by multiple gene variants and environmental factors (particularly those experienced during childhood like nutrition, duration of sleep and stress). Accordingly, adult height within any population is spread out over a continuum, the shape of which is called the 'normal' or 'bell-shaped' distribution. In a similar way, blood sugar levels within a population also follow a continuum and normal distribution. Like height, there are multiple genetic and environmental factors that influence our blood sugar levels at any given moment. In these scenarios in which a condition is defined by a continuous variable, it is common for a 'line in the sand' to be drawn. T2D is one example, in which a vertical line is drawn towards the right-hand side of the normal distribution of blood glucose readings (nominally 48 mmol/mol for HbA1C, an average measure of blood glucose readings over the preceding 3 months), with any reading to the right of which defining T2D. (There are multiple sub-types of Diabetes Mellitus beyond T2D, and diagnosis of each subtype often requires other tests, but T2D is used as an example here as it is the commonest form of Diabetes Mellitus). As a scientist, I never find such 'line in the sand' definitions of disease particularly satisfying or convincing, and there is always the potential to shift the line over time (as indeed has happened on multiple occasions in the past for T2D). Diagnosing such 'continuum' conditions can sometimes feel like placing one's hand on a kettle once filled with cold water, switching it on and being asked to say at which point the kettle becomes hot. (For health and safety reasons, it is probably better that you don't try this at home!).

This is all a long preamble to defining obesity. As a complex condition, obesity manifests clinically on a continuum and therefore suffers from 'line in the sand' mentality. BMI is a globally recognised criterion to define obesity. BMI is a measure of body weight according to height and does have utility on a population level. Like height, BMI within any population follows a normal distribution, and as with T2D, we use a 'line in the sand' to define obesity in any individual. Nominally, a BMI of 30 $kg\,m^{-2}$ or above defines obesity, with lower cut-offs for some ethnic minority groups (*fig 1.3*). The fact that our definition of obesity is bang on 30 $kg\,m^{-2}$ and not 29.56158 $kg\,m^{-2}$ tells us something important: that this cut-off is not scientifically determined, but rather tidily makes use

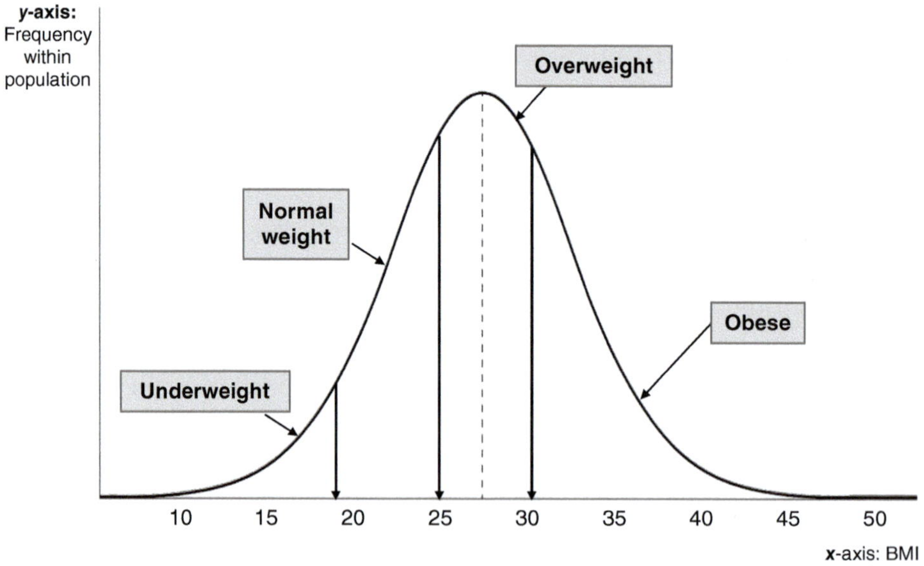

Figure 1.3: 'Normal' distribution of BMI within a population. BMI: Body Mass Index. This is a schematic representation of BMI within a typical western population. Each population varies regarding the precise positioning of the normal distribution along the x-axis, and this positioning within each population also varies over time. The BMI cut-offs shown here relate to a Caucasian white population. For some ethnic minority groups, the BMI cut-offs for overweight and obesity are lower than those shown here.

of our decimal system with a nice round number. As a scientist, this does not sit well with me. In Chapter 3, I discuss the many flaws of BMI when applied at an individual level and the challenges of defining obesity based on BMI.

There have been attempts to devise more sophisticated definitions of obesity, but despite these, BMI continues to predominate. In reality, obesity consists of multiple distinct phenotypic subtypes across body composition, insulin sensitivity, physical fitness, glycaemia and cardiovascular risk (9). We need a more sophisticated and individualised approach to defining obesity in all its varied forms that takes account of the multiple and varied anthropometric and physiological scenarios outlined above, progression of body weight and composition over time (rather than just a snapshot of BMI) and a measure of obesity-related cardiometabolic status. Until then, any attempt at defining obesity will be hampered.

The Origin of Obesity: What Has Caused the Global Obesity Problem?

The global obesity problem cannot be attributed to a single factor. The problem is complex. However, we can say with certainty that our underlying genetic make-up is an important contributor. Why do I say this? There is a term in genetics called 'heritability', which refers to the predictability of transmission of biological traits from parent to offspring (2). Heritability is usually (but not always) mediated by 'heredity', which is the transmission of genetic variants from parent to offspring. Put simply, heritability refers to the extent to which any biological trait is inherited (usually genetically) from parents. If a trait has 100% heritability, this means that all its variability is mediated by biological traits inherited parentally (usually genetically), with no involvement of environmental factors. Although not at 100%, we could say that the heritability of eye colour is close to 100% and of all biological traits is perhaps as close as we can get to a biological trait being completely inherited from our biological parents with very minimal impact from environmental factors. In comparison, we know from multiple reported twin-based studies that the heritability of BMI is between 40% and 50% (8) and maybe up to 60–80% in the subgroup of people living with obesity (8). What this means in practical terms is that for any individual, including you and me, our BMI within our population is largely driven by biological (including genetic) traits inherited from our parents, which in the case of those of us living with obesity, accounts for the lion's share of where your BMI sits on the normal distribution. Just read that sentence again. How many times have you heard the media talk about obesity as an inherited and genetic condition? Even highly esteemed groups, governments and healthcare regulators around the world still consider obesity as a 'lifestyle choice' with no mention of genetics or heritability, when the evidence is staring us in the face. Put another way, blaming someone for developing obesity because of their lifestyle choices is as inappropriate and nonsensical as blaming someone for being taller than 6 feet because of their lifestyle choices. Our adult height and BMI are both heavily influenced by our underlying genetic architecture. When you think about it, if obesity was a lifestyle choice, then you would expect a bimodal distribution of BMI throughout the population, with one peak on the right side of the graph denoting those of us who have 'chosen' to become obese and another peak on the left side for those of us who have 'chosen' to have a healthy weight (*fig 1.4*). This notion, of course, is preposterous, and we only need to look at the distribution of BMI within any population to see that it is normal rather than bimodal and therefore redolent of a biological trait rather than a manifestation of our individual decisions and our conscious choice. Suggesting that obesity is a lifestyle choice, in my view, is shameful and ignorant in equal measure.

Having established the high heritability of BMI, the next question is what gene variants influence our BMI? This is an ongoing and active

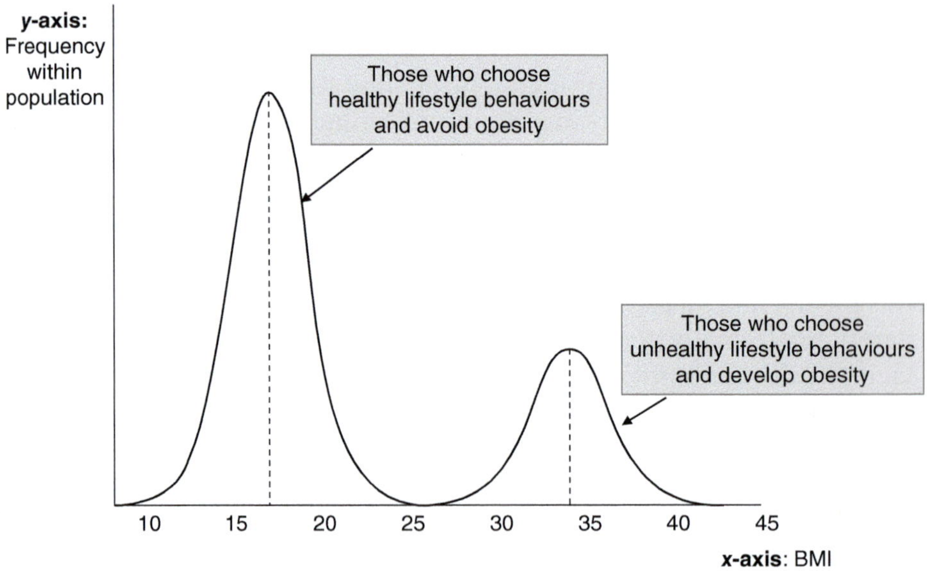

Figure 1.4: Imaginative bimodal distribution of BMI within a population if obesity was a lifestyle choice. BMI: Body Mass Index. This is an imaginative schematic illustration of the type of bimodal distribution of BMI within a population that would occur if obesity was a lifestyle choice: if each of us made a conscious choice regarding engagement in lifestyle behaviours (including dietary behaviours) that contribute to weight gain. We never see this type of distribution of BMI in any population, and the purpose of showing this figure is to illustrate that the widespread misconception of obesity being a lifestyle choice is preposterous and wrong.

field of research, and there have been reported numerous 'genome-wide association studies' (GWAS) that have identified >1,000 gene variants that impact on BMI (8, 10). Although the effect of each individual gene variant on BMI is quite small, it is the cumulative effect of all the variants that have an appreciable effect on differences in BMI between individuals. Imagine a one-arm bandit machine of the type you see at funfairs, but instead of just 3 rows, it contains >1,000 rows, and at the point of conception, this arm is pulled, and what then shows up on the screen will predetermine your individual positioning on the population-wide BMI normal distribution. Of course, the potential outcomes from this thought experiment are determined by the genetics of your parents and more specifically the sperm and egg that formed you. You may be wondering about the function of these many gene variants that influence BMI. This is subject to ongoing research. However, we know that the majority are expressed within the brain and particularly within the hypothalamus that regulates the control of appetite and metabolism (11). (In Chapter 2, I discuss the control of appetite in detail.) In essence, the control switches that determine our appetite and metabolism are set at slightly different levels between individuals, and this then mediates differences in BMI within the population. There are other gene variants that impact on fat distribution, expressed within the fat tissue (11).

Interestingly, despite the GWAS data reported to date on tens of thousands of participants, we have only identified <10% of the genetic variants that account for the overall heritability of BMI. As I intimated earlier, heritability refers to the transmission of biological traits between generations. Whilst genetics is an important contributor to heritability, there may be other factors like 'epigenetics', for example. Epigenetics refers to how genes are expressed rather than to gene mutations or variants. Our genes are made of DNA which is packaged around proteins called 'histones'. Chemical modifications of these histones (like 'methylation' and 'acetylation') influence how tightly our DNA at each location of the genome is wound around each histone protein. This in turn influences the level of expression of each gene. These epigenetic chemical modifications are highly variable between individuals and over time. One useful analogy is to imagine the apps on your electronic device. Think of each app like a separate gene. The app itself may be faulty, analogous to a gene mutation. More likely, there may be some apps on your device that you rarely use and others that you use frequently. In this sense, you are acting like the epigenetic modifications that control your gene expression, through deciding which apps to use at any given time. Just like your choice of app usage may change over time, so too does epigenetic control of your gene expression change over time and responds to environmental and lifestyle changes.

Recent studies have revolutionised our understanding of how epigenetics can impact the transmission of biological traits between generations. Put simply, when we are conceived, we do not just inherit the hardwired DNA (genes) from each biological parent. We also inherit the chemical modifications of the histones that attach to those genes that influence gene expression. In addition, during our development *in utero*, our epigenetics is further influenced by maternal factors, including the environment experienced by our mothers. It seems likely that some of the heritability of BMI is mediated by epigenetic factors and identifying these factors will be a challenge for the future. In addition, our BMI is likely influenced by our gut microbiota (which I discuss in detail in Chapter 5), which itself is subject to trans-generational transmissible mutability between mother and newborn (2). During vaginal delivery, there is oral exposure of the newborn to the maternal gut microbiome (12), which results in greater overall diversity and colonisation of the infant gut microbiota during the first 3 months of life, compared with newborns born via Caesarean section (C-section) (13). Furthermore, maternally derived gut microbes within the newborn gut tend to have a permanence that can last into adulthood (14). Finally, the infant gut microbiota is influenced heavily by human breast milk (which I discuss in more detail in Chapter 5). Although human breast milk is traditionally considered sterile, it is now widely accepted to contain an abundance of diverse microorganisms, translocated from the mother's own gut microbiota (15, 16). In this way, the maternal gut microbiota colonises the breastfed infant gut and facilitates the establishment of the infant gut microbiota (15, 17).

At this point, I can hear you shout 'hang on, wait a minute! What about fast food, unhealthy diets, and reduced physical activity, the usual obesity suspects?' Well, you are correct! The genetic data outlined here provides an insight into the susceptibility of each of us to weight gain and obesity. However, it is also true that our genetics have not really changed for tens of thousands of years and certainly not in the last 50 years! It follows therefore that the global obesity problem has been catalysed by environmental (rather than genetic) changes: sometimes referred to as the 'obesogenic environment'. However, this in no way diminishes or downplays our discussion on the role of genetics in determining our BMI. There are two factors at play. Our genetics determines where we sit on the normal distribution of BMI within our population. It is our environment though that determines the position of the normal distribution of BMI on the *x*-axis. What has happened in the last 50 years is that the entire normal distribution of BMI within our population has shifted to the right, and it is this environmentally induced rightward shift of BMI distribution that underlies the global obesity problem (*fig 1.5*). Ultimately, there are complex interlinks between our genetic architecture and our

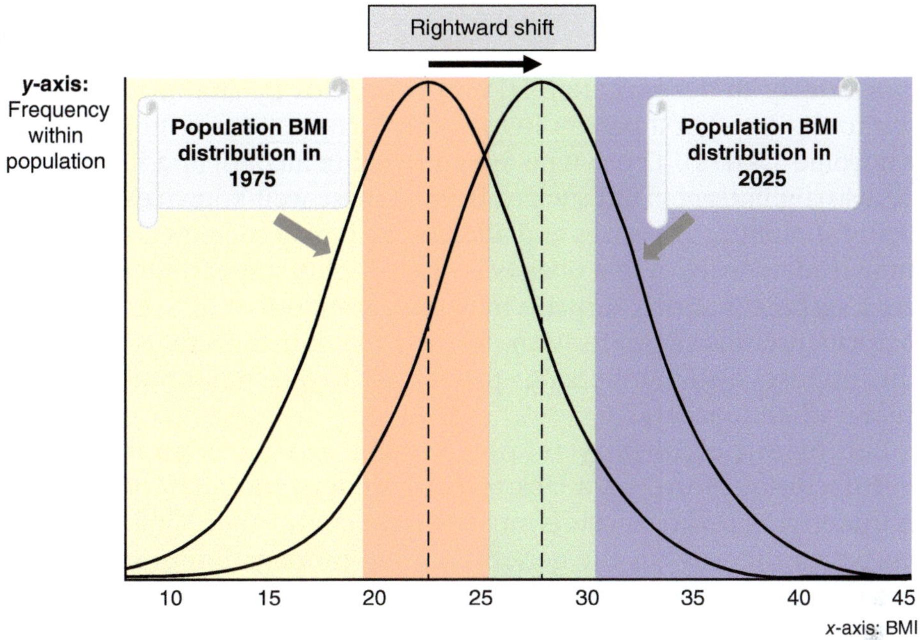

Figure 1.5: Comparison of 'normal' distribution of BMI within the UK population between 1975 and 2025 showing a 'rightward shift'. Schematic representation of BMI within the UK population showing a rightward shift over a 50-year period from 1975 at the start of the global obesity problem, and 2025. BMI: Body Mass Index. The yellow bar denotes underweight (BMI <18.5 $kg\,m^{-2}$); the pink bar denotes normal weight (BMI 18.5–24.9 $kg\,m^{-2}$); the green bar denotes overweight (BMI 25–29.9 $kg\,m^{-2}$); the purple bar denotes obesity (BMI ≥30 $kg\,m^{-2}$). These BMI cut-offs shown here relate to a Caucasian white population. For some ethnic minority groups, the BMI cut-offs for overweight and obesity are lower than those shown here.

environment, and living in an obesogenic environment can amplify our genetic risk of developing obesity (11). I will leave our discussion on environmental factors for now, and return to it in Chapter 12, where I will discuss how we can optimise our future environments to mitigate against weight gain and improve our health and well-being.

The Stigmatisation of Obesity

'Stigma' originates from ancient Greece and referred to a physical mark on the body used to identify criminals, slaves and traitors, intended to shame and ostracise those individuals. Today, stigma refers to a negative perception, disapproval or discrimination against individuals or groups based on certain characteristics and attributes. There are different forms of stigma (including personalised stigma, which is the internalisation of societal stigmatised views), and unfortunate consequences include social isolation, rejection and discrimination. Within medicine, there are numerous examples of stigmatised conditions. Historical examples include diseases like leprosy and more recently those who have contracted Human Immunodeficiency Virus (HIV). Lady Diana famously helped enormously to destigmatise HIV in the 1980s by shaking the hand (without gloves) of a person living with 'Acquired Immunodeficiency Syndrome' (AIDS). Those who are addicted to alcohol and illicit drugs are also stigmatised in our society. Beyond these well-known examples of highly stigmatised diseases and addictions, it may come as a surprise to some readers to learn that obesity is also a highly stigmatised disease (2, 18). I suspect that this surprise may stem from our ability, as a society, to normalise this stigmatisation in a way that blinds us to its existence. This mindset also hampers our propensity to question obesity-related stigma when it occurs.

The origin of obesity-related stigmatisation is complex and multifactorial. However, a lack of basic understanding of obesity and its underlying pathogenesis is an important contributor. This ignorance has paved the way for the generation and propagation of myths and misconceptions (19), which as humans we seem happier to accept and believe rather than live with uncertainty and unknowns (20). Human history is littered with such scenarios: take witch hunts, for example. The media and even governments and healthcare regulators have contributed towards the stigmatisation of obesity, with its portrayal as a lifestyle choice, and reluctance to label obesity as a disease. (In the United States, obesity has been officially recognised as a disease since 2013, and other governments, including the UK government should follow suit.) Through a flawed belief that we can all control our own appetite consciously and choose whether or not to become obese (21), the corollary is an implicit assumption that weight gain and obesity result from a wilful allowance of one's own appetite to control our eating-related behaviours, through vices like greed and gluttony, compounded by laziness and an unwillingness to engage in physical exercise and activity (2). This is a common myth that is widespread within our society (22).

As with so much of human psychology and our psychosocial interactions, much of our stigmatisation of obesity is not necessarily explicit and often operates below our conscious awareness. In one of my first engagements with the national media in the United Kingdom, I conducted an interview with a journalist on Polycystic Ovary Syndrome (PCOS, recently re-named as 'Polyendocrine Metabolic Ovarian Syndrome', PMOS), a common condition in women which also associates with obesity. Unbeknownst to me, the journalist accompanied the article with a highly stigmatised and depersonalised image of female obesity. At the time, I was junior and didn't really question it. Now though, I look back at it in horror. Whenever obesity is portrayed in the media, this is often accompanied by highly stigmatised imagery, promulgating our false beliefs regarding the origins of obesity, sometimes showing a person (often depersonalised) living with obesity and wilfully eating unhealthy doughnuts for example or lounging on the couch. As if to say, 'it is their fault that they are obese, as they have brought it upon themselves through wilfully engaging in such unhealthy lifestyles, and this is so shameful that we are not even going to show the identity of the person'. This is unacceptable! Society needs to look at itself and see this for what it is, which is a form of discrimination, and promulgation of highly stigmatised views. The widespread stigmatisation and discrimination outlined here have contributed towards a dispassionate approach towards those living with obesity (18). This in turn has fuelled a long-term lack of funding to support those living with obesity and to implement strategies for its effective management.

To be clear, I am not blaming journalists or the media for the stigmatisation of obesity. Like you and me, journalists live in the same society and are influenced by the same beliefs and norms. We shouldn't expect our journalists to be saints as much as anyone else in society. I use the example of journalists as their work is there for all of us to see and is a useful mirror on societal beliefs and attitudes. In the context of obesity, this mirror reflects a sick (or at least ignorant) society. Nor do I necessarily blame society. It is important though that we are aware of such stigma and that we strive to address and ultimately eliminate it. Indeed, one of the drivers for me writing this book was to address societal ignorance regarding obesity, to dispel widely held myths and misconceptions and to educate the populace regarding obesity. I accept that to change societal views on any topic is a big task and may take a generation to achieve. Alternatively, there may be a tipping point, which catalyses a sea change in people's attitudes and beliefs towards people living with obesity. Either way, it is important that we address the stigmatisation of obesity across the whole of society, including in our schools, where stigmatised views and attitudes often develop. It is incumbent upon all of us to act. Improved public education and understanding of obesity (including an appreciation of the genetic predisposition to obesity and our lack of conscious control of our appetite) should help in the de-stigmatisation of obesity (2) and facilitate a new dawn of understanding, support and compassion for those of us living with obesity.

Here endeth the first chapter. I hope this has whetted your appetite for more. If so, that's great because that is the focus of the next chapter.

'If music be the food of love, play on...'

(Shakespeare, Twelfth Night).

References

1. World Health Organization. Obesity and Overweight. World Health Organization. 2025.
2. Barber TM, Kabisch S, Pfeiffer AFH, Weickert MO. The gut microbiome as a key determinant of the heritability of body mass index. Nutrients. 2025;17(10):1713.
3. Pi-Sunyer X. The medical risks of obesity. Postgrad Med. 2009;121(6):21–33.
4. Peeters A, Barendregt J, Willekens F, Mackenbach J, Al Mamun A, Bonneux L, et al. Obesity in adulthood and its consequences for life expectancy: a life-table analysis. Ann Intern Med. 2003;138:24–32.
5. Cecchini M. Use of healthcare services and expenditure in the US in 2025: the effect of obesity and morbid obesity. PLoS One. 2018;13(11):e0206703.
6. Nigatu YT, van de Ven HA, van der Klink JJ, Brouwer S, Reijneveld SA, Bultmann U. Overweight, obesity and work functioning: the role of working-time arrangements. Appl Ergon. 2016;52:128–34.
7. Sarwer DB, Polonsky HM. The psychosocial burden of obesity. Endocrinol Metab Clin North Am. 2016;45(3):677–88.
8. Bouchard C. Genetics of obesity: what we have learned over decades of research. Obesity (Silver Spring). 2021;29(5):802–20.
9. Abraham A, Yaghootkar H. Identifying obesity subtypes: a review of studies utilising clinical biomarkers and genetic data. Diabet Med. 2023;40(12):e15226.
10. Loos RJF, Yeo GSH. The genetics of obesity: from discovery to biology. Nat Rev Genet. 2022;23(2):120–33.
11. Goodarzi MO. Genetics of obesity: what genetic association studies have taught us about the biology of obesity and its complications. Lancet Diabetes Endocrinol. 2018;6(3):223–36.
12. Dominguez-Bello MG, Costello EK, Contreras M, Magris M, Hidalgo G, Fierer N, et al. Delivery mode shapes the acquisition and structure of the initial microbiota across multiple body habitats in newborns. Proc Natl Acad Sci USA. 2010;107(26):11971–5.
13. Rutayisire E, Huang K, Liu Y, Tao F. The mode of delivery affects the diversity and colonization pattern of the gut microbiota during the first year of infants' life: a systematic review. BMC Gastroenterol. 2016;16(1):86.
14. Korpela K. Impact of delivery mode on infant gut microbiota. Ann Nutr Metab. 2021;77:11–9.
15. Yi DY, Kim SY. Human breast milk composition and function in human health: from nutritional components to microbiome and microRNAs. Nutrients. 2021;13(9).
16. Togo A, Dufour JC, Lagier JC, Dubourg G, Raoult D, Million M. Repertoire of human breast and milk microbiota: a systematic review. Future Microbiol. 2019;14:623–41.
17. Asnicar F, Manara S, Zolfo M, Truong DT, Scholz M, Armanini F, et al. Studying vertical microbiome transmission from mothers to infants by strain-level metagenomic profiling. mSystems. 2017;2(1):e00164-16.

18. Westbury S, Oyebode O, van Rens T, Barber TM. Obesity stigma: causes, consequences, and potential solutions. Curr Obes Rep. 2023;12(1):10–23.
19. Das B, Khan OA. The myths of obesity. Int J Surg. 2019;68:114–6.
20. Lim JB, Oppenheimer DM. Explanatory preferences for complexity matching. PLoS One. 2020;15(4):e0230929.
21. Mazonde N, Goldstein S. Online health communities' portrayal of obesity on social media platforms in South Africa. J Health Commun. 2023; 28(sup2):15–24.
22. Rubino F, Puhl RM, Cummings DE, Eckel RH, Ryan DH, Mechanick JI, et al. Joint international consensus statement for ending stigma of obesity. Nat Med. 2020;26(4):485–97.

2 Appetite

'Thou canst not speak of that thou dost not feel' is a line from Shakespeare's *Romeo and Juliet*. I think this would also apply if we replaced 'speak' with 'act'. Why do we act in the ways that we do? What drives our behaviour? These are deep questions that have occupied the minds of philosophers, neuroscientists and psychologists for a long time. The answer, as you would expect, is complex with multiple facets. We all behave in the ways that we do for a hundred reasons that include our underlying genetic makeup, our upbringing and past experiences, our hormonal status, our personality, our emotional state at any given time, our personal circumstances and our immediate environment with its many challenges, hazards and opportunities. Amongst this milieu of factors that influence our behaviour looms an important biological phenomenon that we call 'appetite'.

There are multiple forms of appetite. In its broader sense, appetite evolved to drive our behaviour towards certain biological goals. In the reproductive sense there is, of course, sexual appetite. Most other forms of appetite though focus on our survival. The drive to keep ourselves well hydrated, termed 'thirst', is in fact a form of appetite, driving us to drink fluids when we feel thirsty. We all have an appetite to find shelter to protect us from the elements. This drives us to seek appropriate accommodation. We all have an appetite to sleep when we feel tired, and this helps to drive our sleep-wake cycle. The drive to eat food when we feel hungry is just one form of biological appetite, but it is the one that we usually refer to as appetite colloquially: if we say that someone has a big appetite, we usually mean that they have a big appetite for food. In this chapter, I will focus on this form of appetite, the one that drives us to eat. I will explore the underlying neurobiology of appetite and the multiple biological signals that influence our appetitive control, both from the periphery and from other parts of the brain. I will discuss how our underlying genetics influences our appetite in subtle ways and how this influences our overall Body Mass Index (BMI). I will discuss the influence on our drive to eat by factors that extend well beyond our appetite centre, including hedonic (pleasurable) effects from food, and social cues. Finally, I will discuss how our appetite changes when we lose weight and the challenges this creates for the maintenance of body weight and avoidance of body weight regain in these scenarios.

The Neurobiology of Appetite

In the 21st century, there has been a transformation in our understanding of the neurobiology of appetite. These renewed insights stem primarily from rodent-based studies. Control of our appetite occurs within the hypothalamus, a region that sits at the base of the brain. The hypothalamus is about the size of an almond and is a vital structure that controls homeostatic aspects of our biology: this means keeping things on the strait and narrow, including our body temperature and the concentration (osmolality) of our blood. The hypothalamus also controls homeostasis of body weight through changes in our appetite and metabolic rate. The appetite centre resides within a region of the hypothalamus called the 'arcuate nucleus'.

To avoid too much technical jargon, I am going to simplify my explanation of appetite control. One key concept is that rather than a switch that you turn on or off (all or nothing), the control of appetite is through a dimmer switch. This means that the biological control of appetite sits on a spectrum. We can all relate to this anecdotally and think of times when we are extremely hungry, when we could eat a horse and our drive to eat is intense, compared with times when we just feel a little bit hungry, where we may or may not choose to eat something, and occasionally when just the thought of food makes us want to vomit. It is a bit more complicated than this, as in reality, we each have two dimmer switches controlling our appetite: one which steadily increases our appetite ('up-switch') and one which steadily reduces our appetite ('down-switch'). Our appetite at any given time is an amalgamation of the status of our two appetite dimmer switches. There are separate pathways that activate our up- and down-switches. The final common pathway is something called the 'melanocortin receptor'. In effect, the stimulation of our melanocortin receptor represents the amalgamation of the outputs of our two appetite switches and determines how satiated (or hungry) we feel at any given time. Our appetite up-switch inhibits the melanocortin receptors (through 'agouti-related peptide') and our appetite down-switch activates the melanocortin receptors (through 'melanocyte-stimulating hormone') (1). Greater activation of our melanocortin receptors results in reduced feelings of hunger (and greater satiation). In addition to appetite, our melanocortin receptors also control our metabolic rate, which has a reciprocal relationship with appetite. This means that when our melanocortin receptors are stimulated, we feel less hungry, but our metabolic rate also increases. Conversely, when there is inhibition of our melanocortin receptors, we feel more hungry,

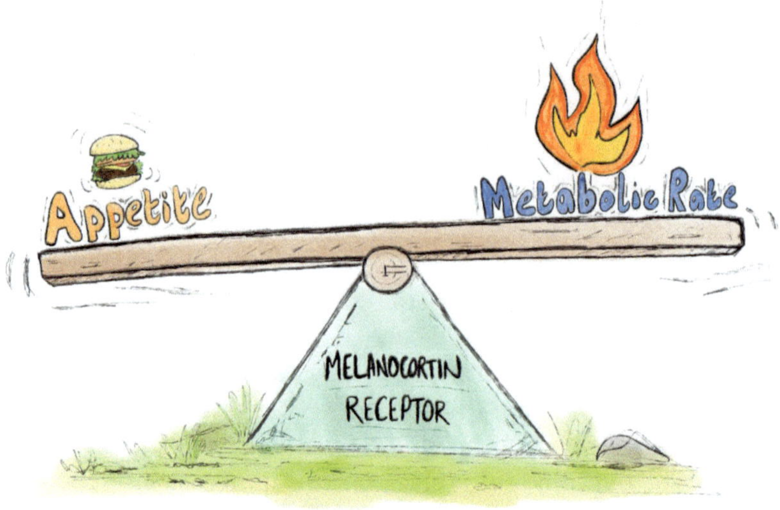

Figure 2.1: The reciprocal variation of appetite and metabolism. The central hypothalamic regulation of appetite occurs through activity at the melanocortin 4 (MC4) receptor, which acts like the fulcrum of a seesaw. When one is up, the other is down, and vice versa.

but there is a reduction in our metabolic rate. Think of hunger and metabolic rate as being at opposite ends of a seesaw: when one is up, the other is down, and vice versa. And the fulcrum is the melanocortin receptor (*fig 2.1*). This is an important point. This insight partly explains why we tend to feel colder when we are hungry: our metabolic rate is lower, and so we are burning off less fuel and generating less heat. Conversely, when we eat food and our appetite becomes satiated, our metabolic rate also increases. This combined with the direct thermic effect of the food in our gut (assuming it was a hot meal), and the thermic effect of the additional metabolism within our liver to help assimilate nutrients after a meal all contribute to feeling warmer after eating a meal.

To simplify things, we can imagine each of our appetite dimmer switches as having a range of values. The up-switch ranges from 0 to +10. The down-switch ranges from 0 to −10. Our appetite at any given time reflects the sum of the values of these two switches. Therefore, when our up-switch is maximally stimulated (+10) and our down-switch is maximally inhibited (0), our appetite is at +10, and we feel extremely hungry. Conversely, when we suffer from gastroenteritis (for example, diarrhoea and vomiting caused by food poisoning) or some other insult to our gut, our up-switch maybe at 0 and our down-switch at −10, and so our appetite is at −10, which makes us feel like vomiting at the thought of food. Most of the time, our appetite is somewhere between these two extremes of +10 and −10 (*fig 2.2*). Physiologically, effects on our appetite dimmer switch often work in tandem and cooperatively. For example,

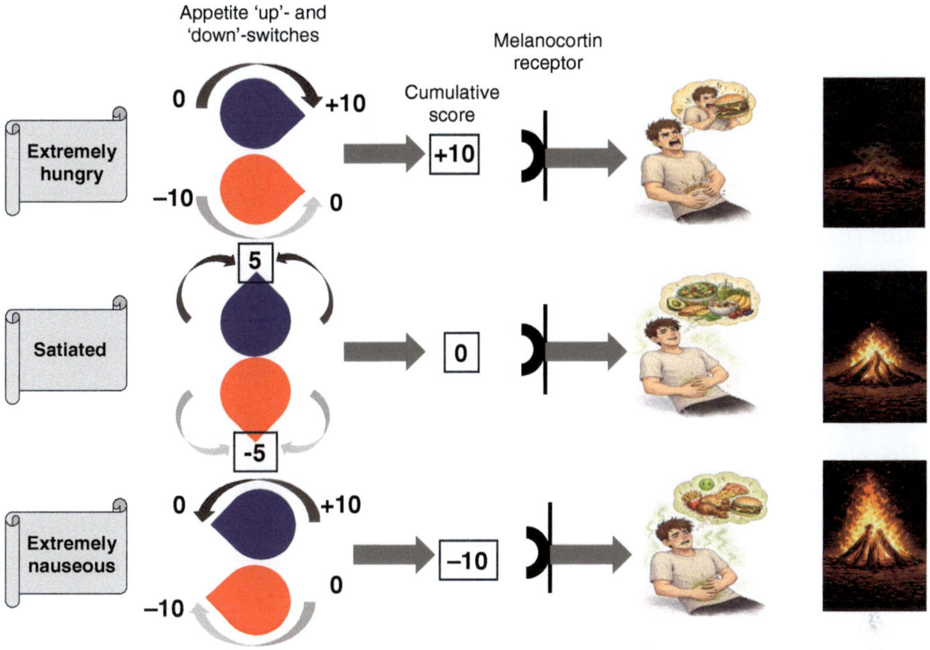

Figure 2.2: Schematic representation of our two appetite dimmer switches and how these influence the regulation of our appetite and metabolism in three scenarios. ('Up-switch' shown in blue; 'Down-switch' shown in red)

leptin, which is an important peripheral signal from fat tissue, acts to stimulate the down-switch and to inhibit the up-switch simultaneously, the cumulative effect of which is to suppress appetite.

That is all you need to know about the neurobiology of appetite. At its very simplest, our appetite is controlled by just two dimmer switches. Rare conditions, caused by single-gene mutations and other chromosomal anomalies, can result in appetite dysregulation. Any interruption to the pathway that controls the down-switch can result in constantly enhanced appetite termed 'hyperphagia'. In our analogy, this is where the down-switch is stuck at (or near) 0, resulting in an unopposed up-switch and with appetite levels constantly above zero. This is the mechanism of hyperphagia for some rare monogenic forms of obesity like 'pro-opiomelanocortin' (POMC) deficiency for example (POMC forms a key component of the appetite down-switch). Similarly, constant over-activity of pathways that control the up-switch can result in it being stuck at (or near) +10, which then overrides any negative signalling from the down-switch, and again with appetite levels constantly above zero. This is one mechanism of hyperphagia in a rare obesity syndrome called 'Prader–Willi Syndrome' (2). Understandably, this constant drive to eat results in weight gain, which often starts in early childhood and can result in extreme forms of obesity. There is also often a diminishment of metabolic rate in these hyperphagic conditions that contributes to overall weight gain (remember the seesaw analogy between the control of appetite and metabolism). Hyperphagia is one of the most unpleasant and troublesome symptoms imaginable, and these patients and their parents, carers and families often experience much distress. Just try to imagine what it would be like to feel ravenously hungry all the time, and regardless of what you eat, you can never properly satiate yourself. You are constantly on the look out for food, even to the point of searching through bins for food that has been thrown-out, or when there is no food around you resort to eating inedible items like cardboard (3). This is no exaggeration. For those who believe in the conscious control of appetite, you only need to look at the extreme eating behaviours of those who suffer from these rare conditions in which hyperphagia manifests. We can no more consciously control our appetite for food as we can resist drinking water when we feel thirsty or we can avoid taking a breath when starved of oxygen. We would be fooling ourselves to think otherwise, and yet so many of us do!

What Controls the Appetite Dimmer Switches?

The two dimmer switches in the hypothalamic appetite centre do not just exist in isolation. There are myriad signals in multiple different forms that influence the status of our dimmer switches and determine the level of our appetite (from +10 to −10) at any given time. These signals are often hormones released from peripheral tissues that travel in the blood before acting directly on the appetite switches. One such hormone, leptin, that I mentioned earlier, is important in the control of our appetite and metabolism. Fat tissue produces and releases leptin. With more fat tissue we release more leptin into the blood. The main purpose of leptin is to reassure the brain that the body has adequate amounts of fat reserves and is not in starvation mode. When there is low fat mass, leptin levels are also low, and this is a potent stimulus for activation of the appetite up-switch (turned up) and suppression of the down-switch (turned down). The net result is an enhancement of appetite and a reduced metabolic rate (the latter to conserve the body's fuel reserves). In addition to influencing the control of appetite and metabolism, leptin also impacts on the gonadal (reproductive) axis: leptin levels need to be above a certain level for the gonadal axis to function and for the body to be in 'reproductive mode' (4). Put simply, if you are starving, then sex is the last thing on your mind. Starvation (with low fat reserves and low levels of leptin in the blood) puts the body in full survival mode, an important aspect of which is a strong drive to find and eat food (and a low sex drive). The close relationship between leptin levels and the function of the gonadal axis also explains why in women of reproductive age menstrual periods can become disrupted or even stop if body weight drops too much, and there is a depletion of fat reserves (and therefore a reduction of blood leptin levels below the threshold that allows the reproductive axis to function). This is an evolutionary adaptation to ensure that pregnancy only occurs in a woman who has enough fat reserves to enable the safe completion of pregnancy, lactation and subsequent child-rearing.

Beyond leptin, there are multiple gut-related hormones that influence our appetite dimmer switches. When we eat a meal, the presence of nutrients in the gut results in the release of incretin hormones (discussed in Chapter 10) and other intestinal hormones. These include Glucagon-like Peptide-1 (GLP-1) that travels in the blood. These hormones have multiple effects, but the control of the appetite dimmer switches is one of them. As with leptin, GLP-1 activates the appetite down-switch and inhibits the appetite up-switch concurrently, thereby resulting in reduced appetite. This is one of the reasons why appetite becomes suppressed whilst eating a meal and stops us from overeating. Other hormones released whilst we eat food have similar appetite-suppressant effects to GLP-1, but through different receptors. These include insulin and amylin, both released from the pancreatic β-cells during and following a meal.

In Chapter 5, I discuss the multiple ways in which our gut microbiota can communicate with the brain, and this includes the control of the appetite dimmer switches. The gut microbiota does this through a variety of ways, including through their metabolic by-products that travel in the blood, but also through impacting on nerve impulses within the vagus nerve, which connects the gut with the brain. Nerve signals that originate in other parts of the brain also influence the appetite dimmer switches. Can you remember the last time you suffered pain such as raging toothache and the effect this had on your appetite and desire to eat? Emotions and stress also influence our appetite, although these effects can be more variable between individuals and difficult to predict and seem to be unique to each of us.

This all seems very neat. We have two dimmer switches and multitudinous signals that are vying with each other to control their settings, with some signals having more influence on the dimmer switches than others. (Think of your thermostat switch at home with multiple people in your household all wanting it to be set at a certain level: the final temperature setting chosen might be a compromise or more influenced by one household member who is a bit more dominant than the others perhaps. This analogy is a bit like your appetite dimmer switches being controlled by multiple signals all the time). At this point though, I do need to throw a fly in the ointment. You will remember our earlier discussion in this section on the appetitive effects of leptin. Based on what I said about low leptin levels during starvation and the enhancing effects of this scenario on appetite, you may have assumed that the opposite happens when you gain weight and become obese. This is a logical assumption. Indeed, with increasing weight gain and obesity, leptin levels in the blood do become elevated, and one might expect therefore that this turns the appetite dimmer switches in a way that suppresses appetite. The question then is why is appetite not naturally suppressed when we become obese and why does this not therefore fix the problem of obesity, drive us to eat less food when we gain too much weight to get our body weight back down to normal levels? If only this were the case! Unfortunately, when we gain weight and become obese, we develop something called 'leptin resistance' (5). What this means is that the leptin in our blood becomes less effective at its receptor in obesity. Put simply, in obesity, although there are elevations of leptin levels in the blood, leptin loses its ability to fiddle the appetite dimmer switches in a way that suppresses appetite (and enhances metabolism). Leptin becomes impotent. Paradoxically, this can lead to enhancement of appetite as we gain weight and develop obesity, driving us to eat more and creating a vicious circle (*fig 2.3*). Analogous to leptin, obesity also associates with insulin resistance, which worsens the problem (like leptin, insulin also normally acts to suppress appetite as outlined above). Insulin resistance is also a nexus for multiple other obesity-related metabolic problems. The good news is that both leptin and insulin resistance are reversible not only through effective weight loss but also through the adoption of healthy lifestyle behaviours such as regular physical activity (discussed in Chapter 7). It follows that any management program for obesity should focus on improving leptin and insulin sensitivities to optimise overall metabolic status and to give back power to these molecules to enable them to fiddle our appetite dimmer switches effectively to reduce our appetite. Such improvements to appetite control through enhanced sensitivity to leptin and insulin also enable enhanced metabolic rate (through the 'seesaw' effect discussed earlier). There are also novel pharmacotherapies in development for obesity management such as *Monlunabant* that can improve leptin sensitivity.

How Our Genes Influence Our Appetite and BMI?

In Chapter 1, I discussed obesity as a heritable condition. That is, our genetics determines our BMI to a large extent and much more than what most people think. This leads to the question of how our genetics determines our BMI. The answer is that we do not fully understand how. However, we believe that a large part of the explanation lies within our individual appetite centres. Genome-wide association studies (GWAS)

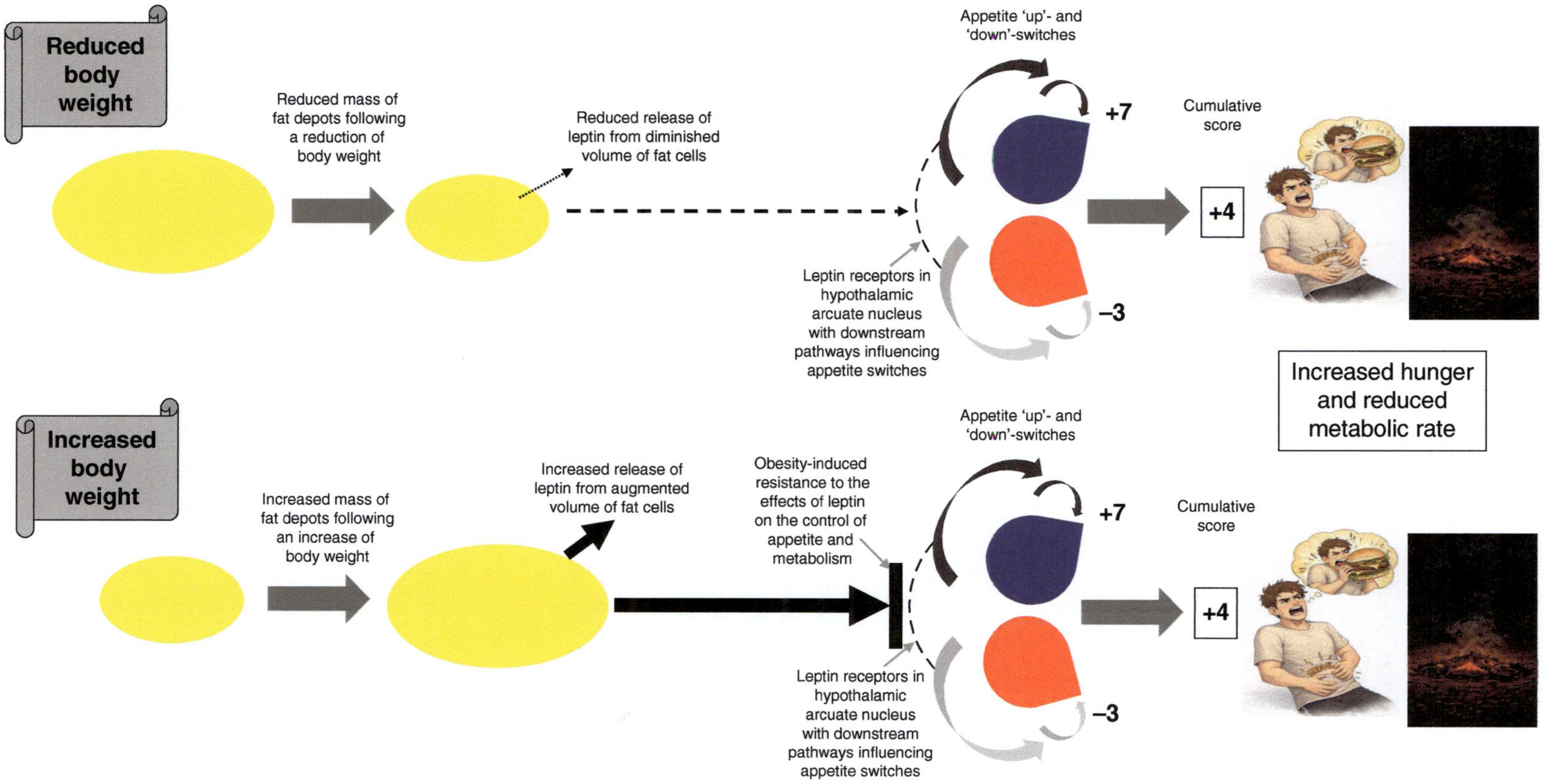

Figure 2.3: The impact of leptin on the position of the appetite switches. ('Up-switch' shown in blue; 'Down-switch' shown in red)

of obesity have identified multiple gene variants that predispose us to weight gain and obesity. The first of these to be identified, variants within the *FTO* gene, influences our body weight by around 3 kg on average: this means that those of us who have one particular variant of the *FTO* gene are, on average, around 3 kg heavier than those of us who have another *FTO* gene variant (6). Further studies reveal that subtle differences in appetite control may account for such differences (7). It turns out that the expression of most gene variants that impact on our body weight occurs within the brain and particularly within the hypothalamic centre that controls the regulation of appetite and metabolism (8). Using our analogy, what this means is that we are all born with slight differences in the settings and ease of movement of our appetite dimmer switches. Some of us are naturally able to suppress our appetite well through a well-oiled switch, whereas in others our dimmer switches may be a little stiff or set slightly too high or slightly too low. We do not fully understand the mechanisms that link our genetics with our appetite control switches. The differences in appetite and metabolic control between each of us are subtle, but they are enough to manifest in discernible differences in body weight, as evidenced by the effects on body weight by the variants of the *FTO* gene. There may be hundreds or even thousands of these gene variants that impact on our central hypothalamic control of appetite and metabolism, and their cumulative effects on the control of appetite and metabolism all add up and determine our overall drive to eat and metabolic rate, and therefore our body weight and propensity to develop obesity.

Whose Appetite Is It Anyway?

As outlined, hunger drives us to eat. The biological control of hunger, through two dimmer switches, is on a continuum, and this is how we experience appetite, with a continuous range of desire for food at any given time. The problem is, as humans, we eat for all kinds of reasons and not just when we feel hungry. Eating is often pleasurable. When we eat, we stimulate the pleasure centres in the brain (including the nucleus accumbens) (1). It follows that we sometimes eat for the hedonic (pleasurable) effects of food. Eating is also a social behaviour, with frequent provision of food at social gatherings. This can be difficult to resist, and we may then eat even when we are not feeling hungry. Another example would be when we feel very cold, we may eat something warm to heat us up again. Therefore, when discussing human appetite and eating behaviour, it is important to understand that this is a complex field. Although the neurobiology of appetite at its core is simple, it can be difficult to discern the determinants of eating behaviours in each of us: that driven by our appetite versus other factors. In Chapter 9, I discuss about the importance of learning to listen to our appetite and how this is a key part of adopting a healthy lifestyle and behaviours.

Appetite as Body Weight Conservator

Homo sapiens evolved over millions of years. This is hard to get your head around, and we are simply incapable of conceptualising such vast timescales. Importantly, our species evolved to survive and to reproduce. Our evolution played out by our distant ancestors on the African savanna. Their highly evolved genetics are what we have inherited. We share the same genetic architecture with our distant ancestors. The problem is that our modern-day obesogenic environment is totally alien to that which our distant ancestors evolved in. Can you imagine any two environments more different than, say, the centre of a mega-city like London and the plains of the African savanna? They may as well be on two different planets (*fig 2.4*). This results in a problem for our modern-day species. The fact is, we are genetic misfits for our modern-day environment.

Starvation would have been one of the biggest threats to the survival of our distant ancestors for aeons. Appetite for food would have developed as a biological countermeasure to starvation: those with a bigger appetite for food would have been more driven to find and eat food and therefore less likely to die from starvation and more likely to reproduce and pass on their genes to the next generation. We can think of this scenario as the evolutionary origin of appetite. Far from it being a problem

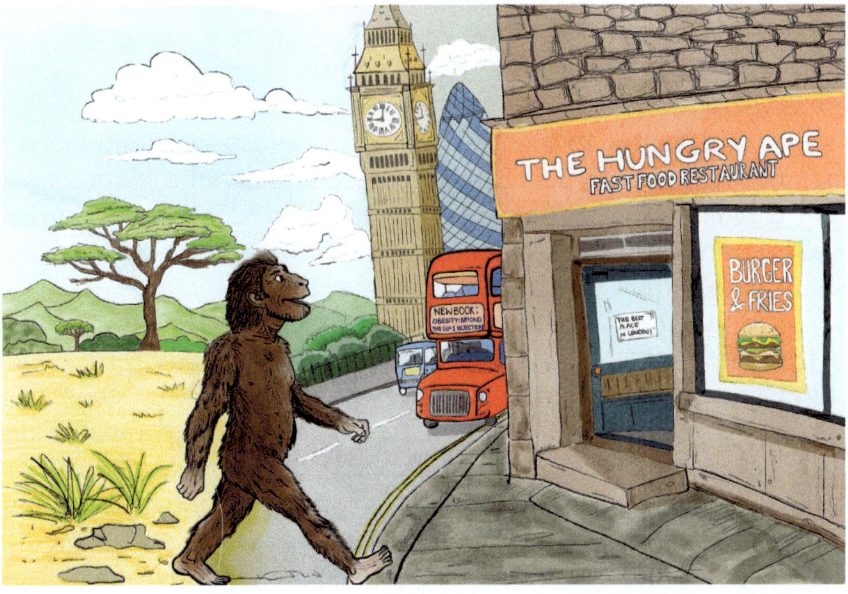

Figure 2.4: What would our hominid ancestors make of our modern-day environment?

for us today, appetite would have been extremely useful to our distant ancestors, helping them to survive. It turns out that there is hardwiring of our biology to protect us from dying from starvation, and this insight is important for our understanding of appetite in our modern-day world.

Earlier in the chapter, I discussed the role of leptin as a hormone that reassures the brain that there is enough fat tissue on board, and this then impacts on the control of appetite and metabolism. In addition to absolute levels of leptin in the blood though, the brain also seems sensitive to any changes to the level of leptin. When we lose weight, our fat mass usually drops, and the level of leptin in the blood therefore also drops proportionately. Even though we may not be starving and our fat reserves may still be good, this drop in blood leptin levels results in a fiddle with the appetite dimmer switches towards enhanced appetite. There are changes in other hormones that affect appetite when we lose weight also, notably ghrelin which comes from the stomach and increases hunger. Studies have revealed that these changes in appetite following weight loss are remarkably persistent and can last at least a year. In addition to changes in the appetite dimmer switches, when we lose weight, there are also changes in the pleasure centres of the brain, which enhance the hedonic effects of food, further driving us to eat. Food tastes and smells better when we have lost weight.

Unfortunately, enhancement of appetite is not the only biological response to weight loss. You will recall from earlier in the chapter that the melanocortin receptors in the arcuate nucleus of the hypothalamus do not just control appetite but also control overall metabolic rate, and the level of our appetite and our overall metabolic rate have a reciprocal relationship like a seesaw. When we lose weight, there is a drop in the leptin levels in our blood. In this scenario, in addition to appetite enhancement, there is also a reduction in our metabolic rate (9). And as with enhanced appetite, this change in metabolic rate is not just transient, but persistent, reflected in its medical term: 'persistent metabolic adaptation' (10). When we lose just 5% of our body weight, there is a reduction in our metabolism, and we can burn off around 100–150 kcal less in each 24-hour period than we did before the weight loss.

It seems that when we lose weight, the body is incredibly conservative and tries very hard to regain that weight. The analogy I use here is to imagine that you are driving a car that is low on fuel. You become super-focused on getting to a filling station: that is the enhanced appetite kicking in. You also drive in a way that conserves your remaining fuel, breaking and accelerating less and switching off the air conditioning perhaps: that is the persistent metabolic adaptation kicking in. The problem with the body's response though is that these persistent appetitive and metabolic adaptations do not just occur when we are running on empty fat stores, but even when there has been a drop in our fat stores when our fat stores remain relatively high (analogous to your car fuel gauge moving from full to 75% full). This is our biological hardwiring, and it is also why >90% of us regain body weight following a reduction in body weight through dieting, for example. If you are one of those, rest assured that you are in a huge majority. And do not let anyone convince you that the reason you regained your body weight is due to personal laziness, greed or any other human form of frailty. This just demonstrates their ignorance. Rather, it is your biology in action. The fact remains that our appetite, along with our metabolism, are conservators of our body weight, and our biology protects us from starvation, but unfortunately not from becoming obese.

I started this chapter with a quote from Shakespeare, and I will finish with more quotes from The Bard. This time from *Julius Caesar*: 'Yond Cassius has a lean and hungry look…', and another from *Henry IV, Part 1*, spoken by Falstaff: 'Thou seest I have more flesh than another man, and therefore more frailty'. There we have it. Insight into the effects of leanness on enhanced appetite, and the health problems linked with obesity, emerging from the works of Shakespeare written over 425 years ago. Prescient indeed!

References

1. Stuber GD, Schwitzgebel VM, Luscher C. The neurobiology of overeating. Neuron. 2025;113(11):1680–93.
2. Kim SJ, Cho SY, Jin DK. Prader-Willi syndrome: an update on obesity and endocrine problems. Ann Pediatr Endocrinol Metab. 2021;26(4):227–36.
3. Bellis SA, Kuhn I, Adams S, Mullarkey L, Holland A. The consequences of hyperphagia in people with Prader-Willi Syndrome: a systematic review of studies of morbidity and mortality. Eur J Med Genet. 2022;65(1):104379.
4. Barber TM, Kyrou I, Kaltsas G, Grossman AB, Randeva HS, Weickert MO. Mechanisms of central hypogonadism. Int J Mol Sci. 2021;22(15):8217.
5. Izquierdo AG, Crujeiras AB, Casanueva FF, Carreira MC. Leptin, obesity, and leptin resistance: where are we 25 years later? Nutrients. 2019;11(11):2704.
6. Cheung MK, Yeo GS. FTO biology and obesity: why do a billion of us weigh 3 kg more? Front Endocrinol (Lausanne). 2011;2:4.
7. Tanofsky-Kraff M, Han JC, Anandalingam K, Shomaker LB, Columbo KM, Wolkoff LE, et al. The FTO gene rs9939609 obesity-risk allele and loss of control over eating. Am J Clin Nutr. 2009;90(6):1483–8.
8. Willer CJ, Speliotes EK, Loos RJ, Li S, Lindgren CM, Heid IM, et al. Six new loci associated with body mass index highlight a neuronal influence on body weight regulation. Nat Genet. 2009;41(1):25–34.
9. Busetto L, Bettini S, Makaronidis J, Roberts CA, Halford JCG, Batterham RL. Mechanisms of weight regain. Eur J Intern Med. 2021;93:3–7.
10. Martins C, Roekenes JA, Rehfeld JF, Hunter GR, Gower BA. Metabolic adaptation is associated with a greater increase in appetite following weight loss: a longitudinal study. Am J Clin Nutr. 2023;118(6):1192–201.

3 Body Mass Index

Imagine you are buying a house. You look on that well-known app that is used widely for this purpose, and you choose a location. But instead of providing you with pictures of each (hopefully well-presented) room and a diagram of the overall layout of the houses in your chosen location, all you get is a list of just two numbers: the height of the house (from ground level to its highest point) and the overall weight (or more correctly, mass) of the house. (Don't ask me how you can accurately weigh a house: that's the beauty of a thought experiment. If Einstein could imagine travelling at light speed, then we can imagine being able to weigh a house: just go with it.) Then imagine that the app churns out a special number for each house called the 'House Mass Index', or 'HMI', which is derived from the mass of the house divided by the square of its height. The purpose of the HMI is to provide you with an indicator of the overall proportions of each house and hopefully reassure you that your future dream home is not a 'slender house' that is 100 feet tall and 3 feet wide and with a very low HMI, or at the other extreme that it is not a troglodytic 'hobbit house' that has an enormous square footage, that is only 3 feet tall and with a very high HMI (*fig 3.1*). Each of these houses may have similar weights but have different HMIs due to their different heights. Now imagine that the value of your chosen house is determined entirely by its HMI, with those houses occupying the 'sweet spot' of perfect proportions between mass and height (this will likely be a range rather than a single value) having the highest value, and those houses outside of this sweet spot range being valued lower, with the 'slender house' and 'hobbit house' being valued the lowest. Importantly, you are blinded to how many rooms your prospective house has and the type of rooms, the state of the plumbing, the electrics, the roofing, insulation and possible subsidence. You don't know whether each room has oak panelling or gold gilding or whether the plaster and brickwork is a complete mess. In fact, you know nothing else about these houses. All those things are irrelevant for the value of your house. All that matters is the HMI and that is all you know. How do you feel about that? Would you go ahead and buy it at auction? I think not.

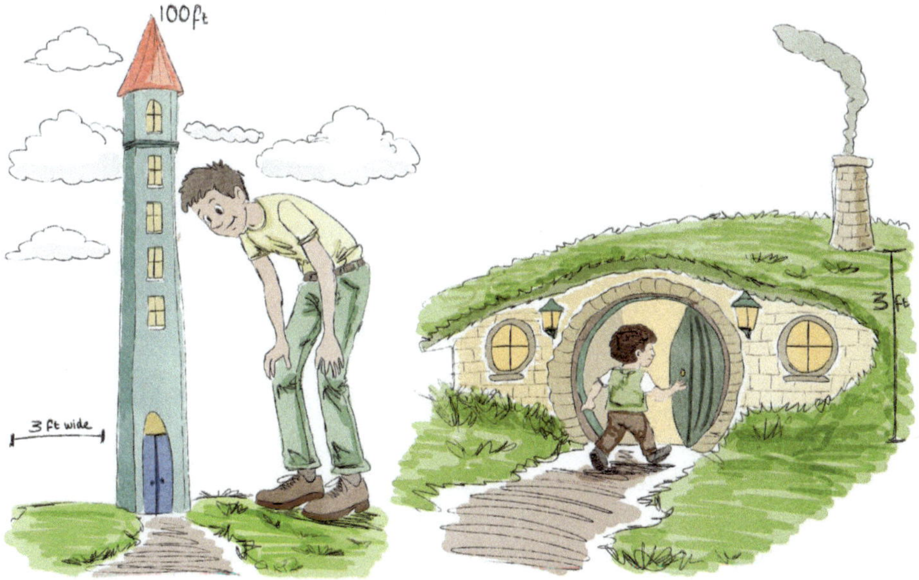

Figure 3.1: 'Slender house' versus 'hobbit house'.

Take that feeling you had at the end of the last paragraph and bottle it. I imagine that it would be one of incredulity, frustration, annoyance and possibly even humour. But more than anything, it would be an overwhelming feeling of wanting to know more. A feeling that there is much more to a house than its HMI, and to buy it you really need to know everything about it, not just its HMI, before reaching deep into your pockets. That feeling you had when reading the last paragraph is redolent of the one that I have, as an obesity expert, regarding the body equivalent of the HMI: 'Body Mass Index', more commonly known simply as 'BMI'. Just like HMI, BMI is also a single number that is derived in a similar way, overall body mass divided by the square of height. Substitute person for house. Also, just like the HMI, BMI is used to make value judgements on people and places us into various ranges, with the sweet spot range being somewhere between 18.5 and 24.9 $kg\,m^{-2}$ and anything outside of that range being considered unfavourable for our health. The further away from the sweet spot range we are, the more unfavourable is our position considered to be and the more we should strive to correct our BMI by getting it more towards (and ideally within) the sweet spot range. It is impossible to write a book on obesity without giving due attention to BMI. Why? Because BMI works its way into pretty much every aspect of obesity. We define obesity by BMI, with an arbitrary cut-off for most of us in the western world at 30 $kg\,m^{-2}$. We define other categories of body status, underweight, normal weight, overweight and various categories of obesity on BMI. We stratify our management approaches to obesity based on BMI (including eligibilities for pharmacotherapies like the GLP-1 injections ['skinny jabs'] or for bariatric surgery). We use BMI to tell us whether we are eligible for infertility treatments, transplant surgery and other procedures. We judge the efficacy of new therapies for obesity based on their ability to improve BMI. And to cap it all, BMI is used and recognised throughout the whole world. It seems that when it comes to all things that are obesity-related, we have a one-tracked BMI-centric mind. Just as with the number of kcals in our food, it seems that we are obsessed with BMI, often to the exclusion of everything else. To use our house analogy, what about the plumbing, the electrics, the roofing and the status of the rooms?

To be clear, I am not suggesting that BMI is a completely useless measure. Quite the opposite. BMI has quite a long history and goes back to the 1830s, when Adolphe Quetelet first proposed the idea. It wasn't called the BMI back then, but rather the 'Quetelet Index' (I suppose you could have guessed this!). In coming up with this index, Quetelet was aiming to define the 'average man' (this was the 1830s, hence the use of the term 'man': nowadays, it would presumably be 'average person'). Crucially though, this index was never intended to be used for the individual, but rather for populations of people, to study how BMI varies throughout a population and to come up with some average measure based on these data. It wasn't until nearly 150 years later, in the 1970s and 1980s (in the early stages of the current global obesity problem), that the Quetelet Index was repurposed as the BMI (1). Even then though, the main purpose of BMI was to describe groups and populations of people, not individuals. On a population level, it is indeed true that there is a broad correlation between BMI and obesity-related comorbidities like Type 2 Diabetes Mellitus (T2D), hypertension (high blood pressure) and obstructive sleep apnoea (2–4). Therefore, as a tool for use in epidemiological studies to define a population, BMI does have some utility. In a similar way, if you were to derive data on the weight and height of all the houses in your country and then group them according to HMI, this would provide quite a useful indicator of how many of them are perfectly proportioned, versus those that are either tending towards slender or hobbit-like proportions, and explore trends of house proportions according to each locality, for example.

One quirky nature of BMI is its use of the squared exponent of height as the denominator. This seems strange as our bodies (and houses) exist in three dimensions, and therefore our body volume should scale with the cubed exponent of height. How this quirk manifests clinically is that BMI can become less accurate at extremes of height (5). The 'ponderal index' uses body mass divided by the cubed exponent of height and so would overcome this problem. The ponderal index is rarely used in clinical practice though. Ponder that!

Beyond this quirk, the main problems with BMI emerge when you try to apply what is, ultimately, an epidemiological population-wide tool to the individual person. In this scenario, two of the main problems with BMI relate to a lack of insight into body composition and body fat distribution.

Body Composition

When you buy a house, its composition is important. You want to know that it doesn't have eight kitchens, no bedroom and no toilet. You want to know how many reception rooms it has, how many bedrooms, how many toilets and whether it has an integral garage. In short, you need to know its composition. As with BMI and the body, the HMI tells us none of these details, and so we are totally blinded, and this can then compromise the utility of the HMI when valuing our prospective future house and considering whether it is the one we want to buy. Imagine Arnold (Arnie) Schwarzenegger in his prime. He would have had a BMI well within the obese range. Armed with just this one measure of BMI, we would assume that Arnie would be at risk for T2D and other obesity-related metabolic problems and may be a candidate for a 'skinny jab' (although they didn't exist when Arnie was in his prime) or even bariatric surgery. We then see Arnie in our clinic and get a shock when we do our physical examination and realise the reason for his elevated BMI is due to the combined weight of his well-developed skeletal muscles (SMs). In fact, nothing about Arnie in his prime would make us think he had obesity. And yet, his BMI would say otherwise.

Body composition does what it says on the tin. In broad terms, the composition of the body means the relative proportions of body weight that comes from fat and lean tissue. The latter is made up from the cumulative weight of our internal organs and our SMs. In each of us, these measures are highly variable due to the individual differences in our fat and SM mass. There are sex differences as well, with women tending to have proportionately more fat tissue and less SM than men, on average. Age differences exist as well, as explained in the next chapter, with SM becoming gradually diminished in its mass as we get older. This is quite a good segue to our next extreme of body habitus, that of an elderly person whom I will call Ernie, with much diminishment in their SM mass (a condition called 'sarcopenia'), in whom fat tissue predominates. Their overall body weight tells us they have a normal BMI, but their body composition may be predominated by fat tissue, putting them at higher cardiometabolic risk. In some sense therefore, we could say that Ernie has a greater candidacy for a diagnosis of obesity than Arnie, despite their respective BMIs suggesting otherwise (*fig 3.2*).

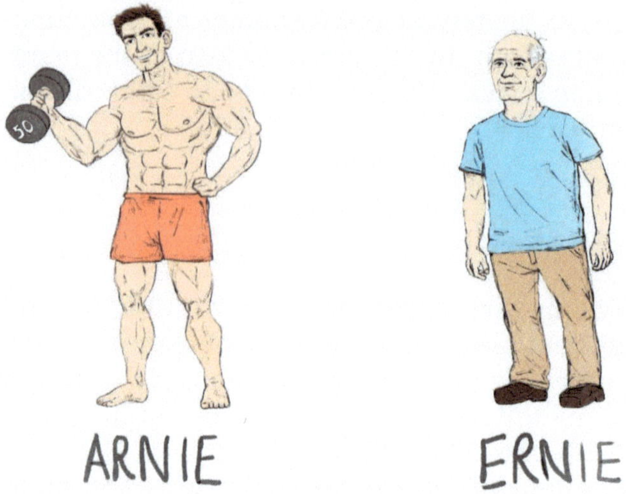

Figure 3.2: Arnie and Ernie.

One of the problems with discussing body composition is that it leads inexorably to a question at the heart of obesity: its definition. (I introduced this topic in Chapter 1.) Yes, our official and globally recognised definition of obesity is based on BMI, but then look at Arnie and Ernie: where do they fit into this scheme?! We need to refine our definition of obesity, but to do this we need to consider carefully what obesity is. This is harder than it sounds. In Chapter 1, I discussed the definition of obesity and used the example of defining an elephant, using descriptive terms. We can all probably agree that on some fundamental level, obesity refers to an excessive amount of fat tissue. It is probably also true that in most cases, excessive fat tissue correlates with an increased BMI. Beyond that, though, we are a bit stuck. There are all kinds of factors that influence the amount of our fat tissue (age and sex, for example), and physiological reasons for why our fat tissue mass may change at certain times (during puberty and pregnancy, for example). Therefore, in each of us, our fat mass is on a trajectory through time and does not normally stay constant. However, unlike BMI, we lack a 'barometer' of our fat mass to tell us what is too much and what is just right at any given time, and for any given individual, this creates a problem.

At its simplest, obesity can perhaps be defined as an excess of fat tissue. Although this is a descriptor, its use here is reasonable as we would normally use the term obesity for anyone with an excessive amount of fat tissue, regardless of its underlying cause. As with BMI though, the problem arises as to how much fat tissue is too much, whether this is different for you and for me and between individuals, and how we ascertain what is a normal amount of fat tissue (and distribution of fat within the body) according to sex, age and other physiological scenarios like puberty, pregnancy, lactation, menopause and the normal ageing process. We simply don't have the answers to these questions. Furthermore, it could be argued that changes in SM mass (as I discuss in Chapter 4) or the emergence of obesity-related metabolic sequelae like insulin resistance should also be included in any future definition of obesity. The fact remains that we really don't have a good definition of obesity. This is a challenge for the future. We can be confident, however, that our current and traditional way of defining obesity as a single disease entity, with its 'one-size-fits-all' approach to diagnosis based on just BMI, is way too simplistic.

Most of us think of obesity as referring to excessive fat tissue. Indeed, the rather pejorative and colloquial descriptive term, 'fat', tells us that. Furthermore, when we use the term 'weight loss' in the context of obesity, what we are usually implying is the loss of fat mass. If you said to Arnie in his prime, 'hey Arnie, you need to lose some weight', this would likely be taken to mean that he needed to lose some of his fat mass rather than to reduce the mass of his SM. Much of the medical literature worsens and promulgates our fixation on overall body weight and BMI (and by implication fat mass), with primary outcome measures of new GLP-1 ('skinny jab') therapies being focused on percentage weight loss, for example. This is often to the exclusion of any focus on changes in body composition. (I am pleased to say that recently, there has been more of a focus on body composition.) The uniqueness of fat mass to each of us as individuals, its variance with age and sex and physiological scenarios and its trajectory over time makes it difficult to pin down as a diagnostic entity. There is a further problem with accurately measuring fat mass. Bioelectrical impedance is an option, but there is controversy in the medical literature regarding its accuracy and reliability. Other imaging techniques like 'Dual-Energy X-ray Absorptiometry' (DEXA) and Magnetic Resonance Imaging (MRI) are too costly and time-consuming to be applicable on a population-wide level.

What about the other component of body composition, SM? I think that SM has been largely forgotten in the context of obesity, eclipsed by its surrounding fat tissue. We are so focused on overall body weight, BMI and fat mass that the demise of our poor SM has remained hidden in plain sight. This is not strictly true as it is often difficult to visualise and examine the SMs in more extreme forms of obesity, precisely because they are hidden from sight by their surrounding excessive fat tissue. In my view, obesity is as much about reduced mass of the SMs as it is about increased mass of fat tissue. In the next chapter, I discuss the importance of SM for our metabolic health and its impact on obesity and the vulnerability of our SMs to reduced mass and function from multiple factors, including excessive fat tissue through crosstalk between each tissue type. It is true therefore that excessive fat tissue tends to associate with reduced SM mass and that obesity can therefore be considered as a metabolic double whammy. An important implication for this insight is that in our management of obesity, we should be as focused on reducing fat mass as we should be on optimising SM mass and function. To summarise, in my view we should redefine obesity as a disease typified by both excessive fat tissue and reduced SM mass and function, each of which contributes independently to adverse metabolic sequelae. This redefinition of obesity gravitates us away from the reduction of BMI and overall body weight as a primary goal of management and towards the optimisation of body composition, with a focus on changes in both fat *and* SM mass. I have suggested an 'adipo-muscle ratio' (AMR) as a useful indicator of body composition (6). The AMR would be a simple ratio between total fat mass and SM mass and could be used to redefine obesity. Use of the AMR would overcome the problems of defining the normality of absolute mass of fat tissue in individuals (for the reasons outlined earlier) but rather would focus on the ratio of each tissue type in individuals (*fig 3.3*). Through considering body composition, the AMR would shift our focus away from total body weight and BMI and instead towards the optimisation of both fat and SM mass in our obesity

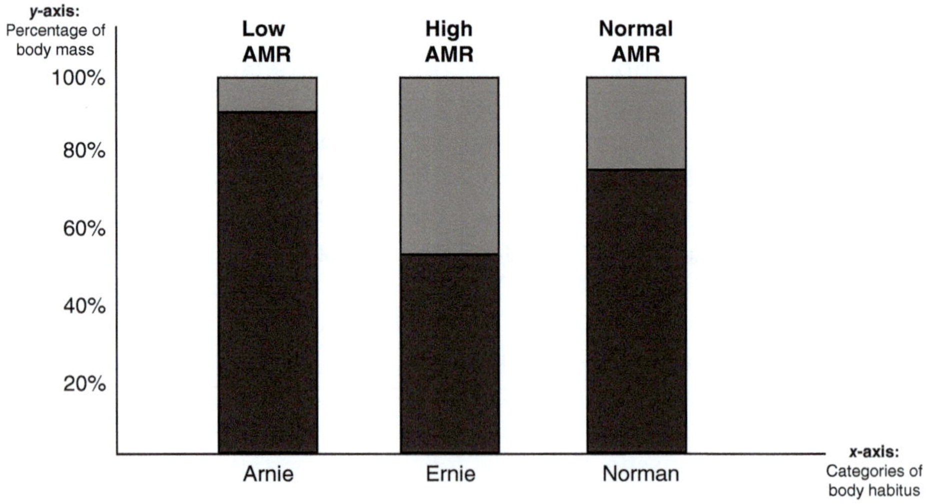

Figure 3.3: Schematic representation of body composition using AMR across variations of body habitus. This schematic illustrates how 'adipo-muscle ratio' (AMR) varies across variations of body habitus. The dark shading represents lean body mass (primarily skeletal muscle [SM]). The light shading represents adipose (fat) tissue mass. In the case of Arnie, he has a very high skeletal muscle mass and a low fat mass, so his AMR is low. In the case of Ernie, he has a low skeletal muscle mass, but a relatively high fat mass, and so his AMR is high. Normal Norman has an average mass of both his lean and fat mass, and so his AMR is normal. This analogy will work equally well for women, although the normal AMR for women is higher than that for men, as women tend to have a higher ratio of fat to lean (including SM) mass than men.

management strategies. Of course, for the AMR to be clinically applicable would require us to develop accurate, reliable, accessible, cheap, non-invasive and widely available biomarkers of total body fat and SM mass: a challenge for the future.

Body Fat Distribution

The main flaw of BMI is its blinding to body composition. In addition, BMI is also blinded to the distribution of body fat. To go back to our house analogy, the HMI tells us nothing about the distribution of the rooms: that the kitchen is on the ground floor rather than in the attic, for example. From a metabolic perspective, body fat distribution is important. Broadly, there are three locations in which fat can be deposited. These include under the skin (subcutaneous), around the abdominal organs (visceral) and around and within organs, including the liver, heart and SM (ectopic). Of these, visceral and ectopic fat are bad news metabolically (7), tend to cause insulin resistance and are a forerunner to T2D and other dysmetabolic conditions. Ectopic fat typically gets deposited when there is an overall excess of body fat mass. Body fat distribution tends to follow sex-specific patterns. Visceral fat (or 'belly' fat around the abdomen) is commoner in men and is sometimes referred to as 'apple-shaped', and subcutaneous fat (particularly around the thighs and buttocks) is commoner in pre-menopausal women and is sometimes referred to as 'pear-shaped' (*fig 3.4*). This is one reason why men tend to have a higher metabolic risk than women (8). The bad

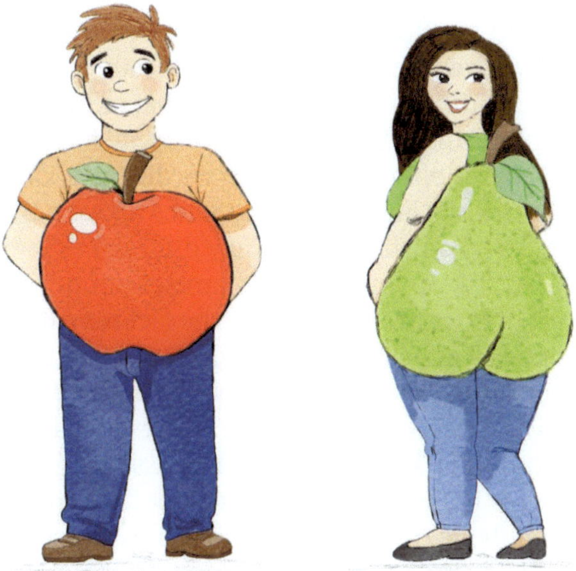

Figure 3.4: Apples versus pears.

news for women is that once past menopause, fat distribution tends to shift towards a more male-like pattern, with more visceral fat.

Beyond the AMR as a measure of body composition, we need an additional measure of body fat distribution to provide insight into overall cardiometabolic risk. It turns out that the waist circumference is quite a good proxy measure of visceral fat and, as crude as it may sound, can provide a useful insight into the metabolic sequelae of obesity. Indeed, waist circumference forms an integral part of the definition of metabolic syndrome (a constellation of obesity-related conditions that increase overall cardiometabolic risk).

When buying a house, there is a long list of factors beyond HMI that need to be considered carefully, such as plumbing, electrics and structural support. Likewise, beyond body composition and body fat distribution, there is quite a long list of other indices that provide insight into the metabolic status of those living with obesity. Some of these go beyond the scope of this chapter. The point to make though is that all these additional indices are blindsided by BMI. I want to give special mention to the inflammatory status of our fat tissue. This might sound strange, but it is not just the amount of fat tissue and its distribution that determines cardiometabolic risk. The status of fat tissue is also important. Sometimes there can be a low-grade inflammatory reaction within peripheral tissues like fat (9), influenced by the status of our gut microbiota (see Chapter 5). In these scenarios, insulin resistance is worsened, and this can be a forerunner for dysmetabolic conditions like T2D (10). Unfortunately, we lack accurate, reliable and non-invasive biomarkers of the inflammatory status of fat tissue, which currently relies upon fat biopsy and visualisation under a microscope.

I have mentioned cardiometabolic risk a few times now. You might be wondering why I keep referring to this. Obesity associates with over 50 weight-related conditions. There is a long list of other obesity-related problems that implicate mental health, psychosocial functioning and work productivity, for example. Why single out cardiometabolic risk? Obesity impacts negatively on our life expectancy. Once above a BMI of 30 $kg\,m^{-2}$ (on a population level) our life expectancy diminishes commensurately. Although increased risk of various malignancies doubtless contributes to this increased risk of premature mortality, the fact remains that cardiovascular events (like heart attacks [or myocardial infarction to give its correct medical name] and strokes) account for the lion's share. Cardiometabolic risk simply refers to the risk of having one of these cardiovascular events. One problem with BMI is that it is not ideal for assessing someone's overall cardiometabolic risk. In my view, any future redefinition of obesity should focus on cardiometabolic risk. AMR and measures of body fat distribution will go some way to achieving this aim. However, it would also be useful to incorporate non-invasive biomarker measures of inflammatory status within fat tissue because of the known association of fat tissue inflammation with increased cardiometabolic risk (10). A further important contributor to overall cardiometabolic risk, worthy of mention, is cardiorespiratory fitness (11) that would also benefit from its own non-invasive biomarker to be used in future clinical (and non-clinical) algorithms.

In short, rather than our current anachronistic and frankly inadequate use of BMI to define all things obesity related, there is an urgent need to improve the utility and clinical meaningfulness of the criteria used to define obesity, on which we stratify and appraise our various management approaches. In my view, a novel approach to obesity definition is required that places emphasis on body composition like the AMR and body fat distribution, in addition to other key measures of obesity-related cardiometabolic health such as fat tissue inflammatory status and cardiorespiratory fitness. Such a shift would help to re-frame the quiddity of obesity, refocus our minds on treatment targets and goals and provide some much-needed logic and fairness regarding how we stratify and prioritize management approaches for those living with obesity. There have been some attempts to redefine obesity, most notably the 'Edmonton Obesity Staging System' that incorporates both obesity-related comorbidities and functional limitations into its definition (12). Furthermore, the 'American Association of Clinical Endocrinologists' published recommendations to recognise a more medically meaningful definition of obesity (13). We need to go further though, and we need international discussion and consensus. We need to transition obesity and its definition into the 21st century. Let's learn some lessons from our imaginary HMI-based house-buying escapades and apply them sensibly to the field of obesity. To boldly go where no one has gone before.

References

1. Health implications of obesity. National Institutes of Health Consensus Development Conference Statement. Ann Intern Med. 1985;103 (6(Pt 2)):1073–7.
2. Chan JM, Rimm EB, Colditz GA, Stampfer MJ, Willett WC. Obesity, fat distribution, and weight gain as risk factors for clinical diabetes in men. Diabetes Care. 1994;17(9):961–9.
3. Sharma AM, Engeli S, Pischon T. New developments in mechanisms of obesity-induced hypertension: role of adipose tissue. Curr Hypertens Rep. 2001;3(2):152–6.
4. Rankinen T, Kim SY, Perusse L, Despres JP, Bouchard C. The prediction of abdominal visceral fat level from body composition and anthropometry: ROC analysis. Int J Obes Relat Metab Disord. 1999;23(8):801–9.
5. Nuttall FQ. Body mass index: obesity, BMI, and health: a critical review. Nutr Today. 2015;50(3):117–28.

6. Barber TM, Kabisch S, Pfeiffer AFH, Weickert MO. Optimised skeletal muscle mass as a key strategy for obesity management. Metabolites. 2025;15(2):85.
7. Goossens GH. The metabolic phenotype in obesity: fat mass, body fat distribution, and adipose tissue function. Obes Facts. 2017;10(3):207–15.
8. Okura T, Nakata Y, Yamabuki K, Tanaka K. Regional body composition changes exhibit opposing effects on coronary heart disease risk factors. Arterioscler Thromb Vasc Biol. 2004;24(5):923–9.
9. Hanson P, Barber TM. Should we use BMI as a selection criterion for bariatric surgery? Expert Rev Endocrinol Metab. 2019;14(4):221–3.
10. Harte AL, Tripathi G, Piya MK, Barber TM, Clapham JC, Al-Daghri N, et al. NFkappaB as a potent regulator of inflammation in human adipose tissue, influenced by depot, adiposity, T2DM status, and TNFalpha. Obesity (Silver Spring). 2013;21(11):2322–30.
11. Ross R, Blair SN, Arena R, Church TS, Despres JP, Franklin BA, et al. Importance of assessing cardiorespiratory fitness in clinical practice: a case for fitness as a clinical vital sign: a scientific statement from the American Heart Association. Circulation. 2016;134(24):e653–e99.
12. Sharma AM, Kushner RF. A proposed clinical staging system for obesity. Int J Obes (Lond). 2009;33(3):289–95.
13. Garvey WT, Garber AJ, Mechanick JI, Bray GA, Dagogo-Jack S, Einhorn D, et al. American association of clinical endocrinologists and American college of endocrinology position statement on the 2014 advanced framework for a new diagnosis of obesity as a chronic disease. Endocr Pract. 2014;20(9):977–89.

4 Muscle and Metabolism

Way back in the early 1990s, I studied Medical Sciences at Cambridge University. During the Anatomy part of the course, I was lucky enough to have been taught by the world-renowned educator and legendary Professor Harold Ellis. During our lecture on the stomach, I recall Professor Ellis's description. He said 'Some people say the stomach is a repository for food. Some people say the stomach is a muscular bag. Yet others say the stomach is a stomach is a stomach!' Those words must have made an impression on me as 30 years later I can still remember them being spoken by the great man. When thinking about any organ in the body, our description of it is heavily influenced by our perspective. For example, whether defining its function or appearance or some other aspect of it. To say the stomach is a muscular bag is entirely correct, because that is what it is. However, I could equally describe the heart as a muscular bag, albeit one with four separate chambers, because that is what it is also. But the stomach and heart of course have entirely different functions, and there are many other ways in which the two organs can be differentiated from one another.

To introduce this chapter, we need to think about the quintessence of a muscle: what it does. To do this, let's have a thought experiment in which you imagine what it would be like to have no muscles at all. For a start, we wouldn't be able to move any of our limbs of our own volition. We wouldn't be able to pump blood around our vessels. We wouldn't be able to move food through our gut through peristalsis, and we wouldn't be able to breathe or blink or speak. When I was at primary school, I played a highly demanding role in one of our theatrical productions, to pose as a tree throughout the entire performance. (I like to think that I was chosen for this role because of my exemplary acting skills, shining through at such a young age.) This is what it would be like to have no muscles. We would become human trees, rooted to the spot, moving only involuntarily with the wind and relying on whatever the atmosphere and soil can provide for us (*fig 4.1*). Thank goodness for muscles!

There are actually numerous benefits of muscles, but they all are defined by one thing: they contract. Through contraction, muscles enable us to be

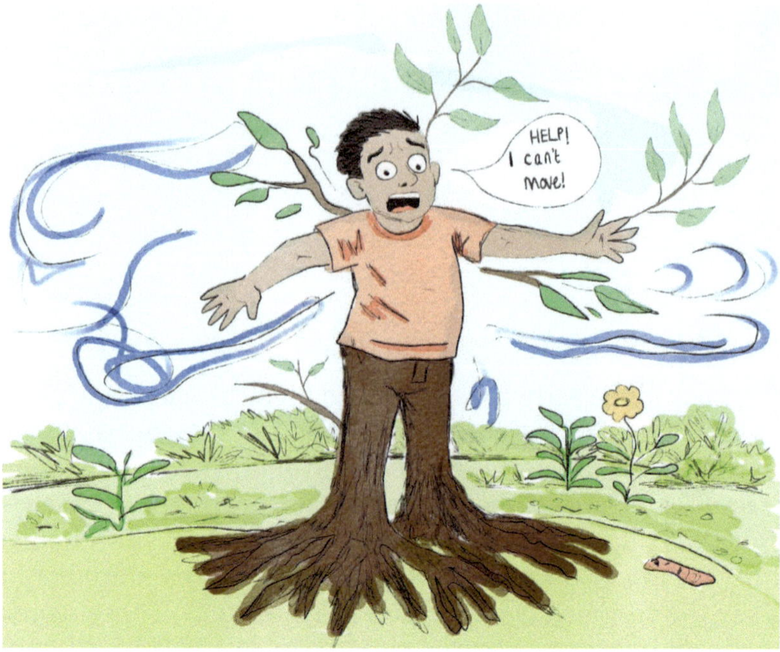

Figure 4.1: The muscleless human tree.

human. There are three types of muscle. Two of them we have already alluded to: 'cardiac' (heart) muscle and 'smooth' muscle, which lines our gut (including stomach) and blood vessels. These two types of muscle are under the control of the body's autopilot system, the 'autonomic nervous system,' which operates without us needing to think about it. The third type of muscle, the 'skeletal' muscle (SM) is the main component of our muscle mass, and it is the SM that we focus on in this chapter. In fact, SM forms the largest organ system in the body, and as such SM contributes a substantial proportion of body composition and weight. SM is composed of the 'sarcomere' (the basic contractile unit) (1). As might be expected, men tend to have a greater proportion of their body weight as SM than women (around 38% versus 31%, respectively) (2). 'Skeletal' just means that these muscles attach themselves to bones within the skeleton through tendons. SM enables us to walk and interact with our environment, through movement of our limbs, hands and fingers. SMs have a vast array of shapes and sizes. The tiny stapedius is the smallest SM in the human body at 1mm in length. The stapedius, by dampening down the vibrations in the middle ear, stops us from deafening ourselves when we talk, shout or sing. In my experience, the stapedius is also a godsend for putting a kibosh on the vibrations elicited within the middle ear when attending a karaoke bar! The biggest SM in the human body is the mighty gluteus maximus within the buttocks, essential for locomotion and beloved of the great renaissance artists Michelangelo and Da Vinci.

Unlike smooth and cardiac muscle, SM is not usually under autopilot, but rather under our own conscious control, and we therefore have volition over our own movements. Complex movements like walking require multiple SMs to contract in a highly ordered, time-dependent and sequential fashion, coordinated through a region of the automated brain called the cerebellum. However, even with walking, we can still choose when to start and stop walking or how fast to walk, even though when we walk, we don't usually have to think about it too much, except, of course, if you are under the influence of alcohol or a member of the 'Ministry of Funny Walks'! Sometimes, SM contracts without our conscious control, such as the knee jerk, the control of which bypasses the brain at the level of the spinal cord. Finally, there is one SM that is vital to our survival: the diaphragm, which marks the boundary between our chest and abdomen, a big dome of muscle that attaches to the lower ribs, and which enables us to breathe. Unusually, the diaphragm is under both autonomic and voluntary control, which is just as well as we need to breathe to survive. There is an awful condition called 'Ondine's curse' in which there is loss of the automated control of the diaphragm (particularly during sleep) and the only way to breathe and to stay alive is through consciously controlling breathing all the time. That is the stuff that nightmares are made of!

To summarise, muscles contract, come in three forms and are either under autonomic and/or voluntary control. The SM enables our limbs to move. SM (particularly those in the back around our spine) are also essential for maintaining posture and help us to prevent falls. Furthermore, SM also protects us from traumatic injury through providing support and shielding for our internal organs. At this point, you might be wondering why I have chosen to include a chapter entirely devoted to the SM and what possible relevance the SM has to obesity. Well, it turns out that the SM has every possible relevance to obesity. Furthermore, there are commonly held misconceptions throughout our society to the contrary. This includes the idea that obesity is all about excessive fat tissue, reflected by the colloquial (and rather offensive) term 'fat'. This misconception is not helped by our reliance on BMI to define obesity and to gauge our success at losing weight (BMI tells us nothing about body composition or about the mass and status of the SM). Furthermore, some of us adopt 'yo-yo dieting' with recurrent cycles of weight loss and weight regain, without appreciating the harmful effect of this approach to our SM. In this chapter, I will discuss what we mean by metabolism and explain why SM plays a central role. I will then discuss the inherent vulnerability of our SM and finally what strategies can be adopted (both now and in the future) to protect our SM, particularly in the context of obesity. In this way, I hope that I will address some of the common misconceptions about SM outlined earlier.

Metabolism

Have you ever noticed what happens to your car engine after a long drive? The heat generated from the engine is a form of metabolism. In fact, whenever energy is converted from one form to another, there is often heat released as a by-product. This is also the reason why our computers (and car engines) need fans to stop the electrical (and mechanical) components from overheating. The human body is no different. Within each of our trillions of cells, there are innumerable processes going on all the time. Compared with the interior of one of our cells, Piccadilly Circus is no comparison! Cells build, fold and package proteins, neutralise harmful toxins and bugs, transcribe our DNA, take in nutrients and transport a myriad of chemicals. All these processes generate tiny amounts of heat (which cumulatively result in our body temperature), proportionate to the amount of work done. This is why we produce more heat and often sweat during physical exercise, due to the increased metabolic demand of our contracting SMs. It is also why we often feel hotter following a meal, as the liver is a metabolically active organ, and needs to work hard after a meal to assimilate the nutrients that are absorbed from the gut. All the processes outlined here define metabolism.

Where does all the energy for these cellular processes come from? Nutrients within our food (mainly carbohydrates and fats) are converted into a molecule called 'Adenosine Triphosphate' (ATP) within the mitochondria (the 'Royal Mint' within the cell). Think of a molecule of ATP as a single Great British Pound coin (actually, the analogy works better if you think of a £1 note, that will be remembered by those readers over a certain age). This is the unit of currency that is used to 'pay' for all the processes going on in our cells all the time. In essence, ATP is broken down within the cell, and the energy released powers everything. One of my favourite facts in biology is that the human body produces its own weight in ATP every single day. For nerds, it is around 1.5×10^{26} molecules of ATP each day. That number is a thousand times larger than the number of stars in the observable universe. Just think about that for a second. 'Ah' I hear you say, 'why is it then that the body doesn't keep doubling its weight every day?' (which in around 43 days would result in you weighing as much as the Earth!). The reason is that the body uses all this ATP every day to power its cells (isn't that incredible!), so there is no *net* change in body weight.

To summarise, each of our cells takes in nutrients from the blood, and some of these are converted to ATP, which is then used as a form of currency to 'pay' for all the processes occurring within our cells. Heat is released in the process. Far from being wasted, this heat helps to maintain a constant body temperature of around 37°C for our cells to work properly and to avoid hypothermia in cold weather. It turns out that some

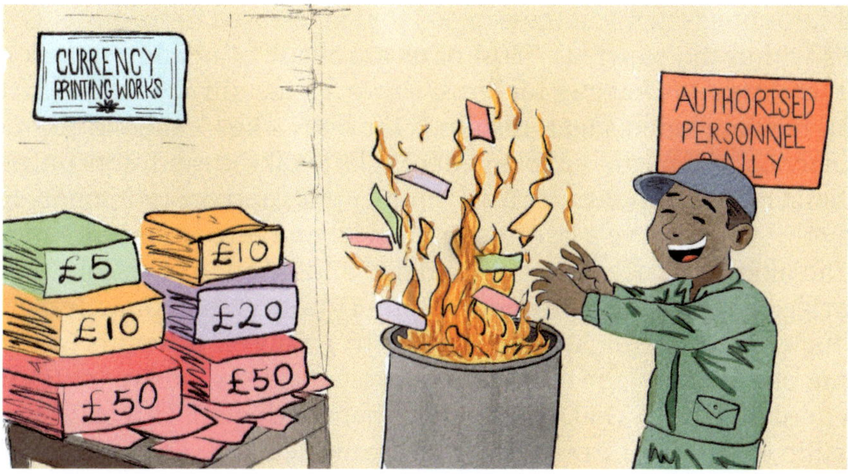

Figure 4.2: The rogue Royal Mint employee.

cells are specialised to produce heat (a process termed 'thermogenesis'). Instead of being converted to ATP, some nutrients are instead just broken down and the energy from their chemical bonds released as heat and 'uncoupled' from the mitochondrial process of generating ATP. Think of a rogue employee in the Royal Mint who just burns the paper supply to keep themselves warm rather than using it to produce banknotes! (*fig 4.2*) It turns out that our SM does exactly that (well, not exactly burning banknote-destined paper that is!). In fact, SM is the largest thermogenic organ in the body and a major contributor to metabolic rate (3). The SM releases heat via the 'SERCA' pump. ('SERCA' is a bit of a mouthful and stands for 'Sarco/Endoplasmic Reticulum Calcium-ATPase'), regulated by a small protein called 'sarcolipin' (3). There are lots of factors (including various hormones and insulin sensitivity) that influence the activity of sarcolipin and therefore how much heat is released from the SM (3, 4). Physical exercise and fitness also influence the activity of sarcolipin, which is one of the many reasons why we should optimise our physical activity. Importantly, for our discussion, the amount or mass of SM has a substantial impact on overall thermogenesis and metabolic rate. Therefore, maintaining good amounts of SM mass helps to mitigate against propensity for weight gain (through heightened metabolic rate).

In addition to thermogenesis, SM also plays a central role in the efficient metabolism of nutrients. When we ingest sugar (carbohydrate), most of it (>80%) gets taken up into the SM (1, 5). Likewise, after a protein meal, much of the amino acid components are also taken up into the SM, which then acts as a reservoir for amino acids that can be released at times of need and even used as an alternate fuel source (6). These processes of carbohydrate and amino acid uptake into the SM following a meal are under the control of insulin, which plays a key role in metabolism. Insulin is a hormone (chemical messenger) that is released from specialised (β) cells within the pancreas. Most of us are aware of insulin (or lack of it) in the context of Diabetes Mellitus. However, insulin does so much more than regulate blood sugar. Insulin is the body's key 'anabolic' hormone. ('Anabolic' just means enablement of cells to take up and store nutrients, to build complex molecules from simpler ones and the promotion of cell growth.) Insulin levels rise after a meal when there are lots of nutrients in the blood that need to be assimilated and taken up into cells. Insulin provides a 'key' for this process to occur. However, sometimes (especially in the context of weight gain and obesity), the cell receptors (or 'locks' using our analogy) for insulin can become less responsive to its effects (in need of some WD40 squirted into them perhaps!). This state, termed 'insulin resistance', forms a nexus for many metabolic diseases, including Type 2 Diabetes Mellitus (T2D). Put simply, the effects of insulin are diminished in obesity, and therefore anabolism is downregulated. Insulin resistance is bad news for the SM, as it results in less carbohydrate (sugar) and amino acids taken up into the SM following a meal, which can contribute towards the development of T2D (1, 7). (More sugar then stays in the blood after a meal contributing to raised blood glucose [sugar] levels). Finally, in addition to the insulin receptors themselves, another important contributor to metabolic efficiency within the SM is simply the amount or mass of SM. A greater amount of SM means a bigger target for insulin and therefore more opportunity to exert its anabolic effects. Reduced SM mass has all kinds of negative implications for metabolism, including reduced uptake of carbohydrate and amino acids into the SM following a meal and reduced thermogenesis, meaning that we burn off fewer calories and become more susceptible to both weight gain and hypothermia (the latter particularly in elderly people). Unfortunately, the SM are vulnerable to diminishment and demise from multiple angles. This forms the focus for the next section.

Cannon to Right of Them, Cannon to Left of Them

Imagine being a SM. You would spend all your life working (well, contracting actually), and all whilst you gradually become smaller, less efficient and weaker. What a terrible demise! It would be a bit like leading the 'Charge of the Light Brigade' by Alfred, Lord Tennyson, with cannons going off all over the place, and your fighting capacity undergoing a gradual process of attrition (*fig 4.3*). From the perspective of a SM, life is certainly not a bed of roses, but rather one of gradual, progressive and inevitable decline and diminishment. In addition to physical weakness, another unfortunate consequence of SM decline is reduced metabolic efficiency. As alluded to in the last section, in this scenario there is increased insulin resistance

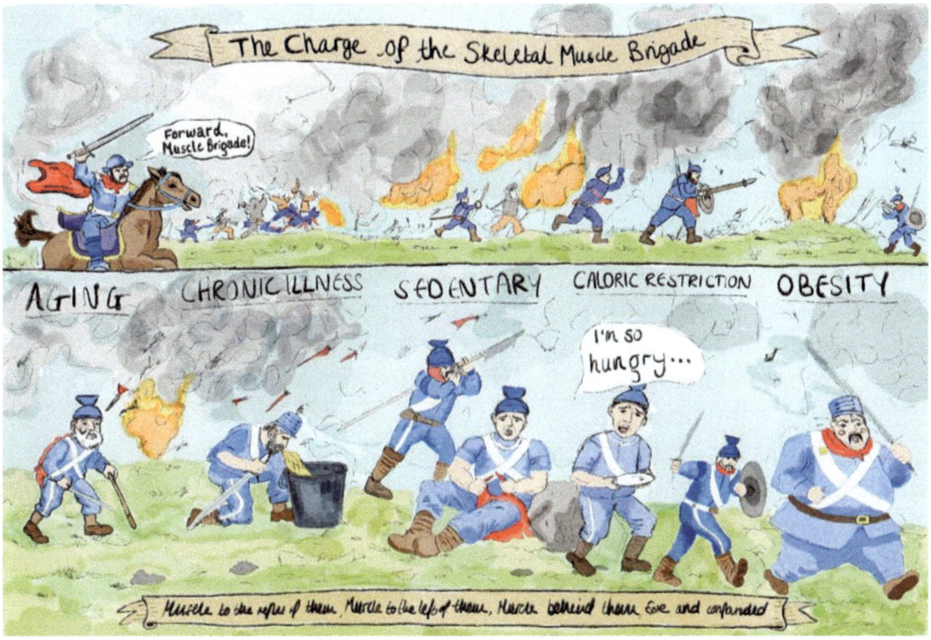

Figure 4.3: The charge of the skeletal muscle brigade.

(a forerunner of many metabolic problems) and impaired thermogenic potential, with implications for reduced metabolic rate and increased propensity for hypothermia (due to our internal 'boiler' not working as well). Diminished SM also typically worsens our quality of life, increases risk of falls and physical disability and delays recovery from illness (6).

The first vulnerability of the SM comes from the normal aging process itself. To use our battle analogy, the longer your army stays on the battlefield, exposed to all the cannons and other weapons, the greater its attrition. All of us age. Like death and taxes, aging is, unfortunately, an inevitability. Admittedly some of us age biologically more rapidly than others, and we should all strive to slow down the aging process through the adoption of a healthy lifestyle. However, whatever we do, aging still occurs. The decline in SM mass is one of the more noticeable effects of aging. This process usually starts in our 20s and often becomes noticeable in our early 50s (1, 2). Over decades, age-related decline in SM mass contributes towards reduced physical strength (ultimately, frailty) and has important implications for global health and economics (8–11).

I can hear you ask, what is it about aging that results in the demise of SM? There are likely numerous contributory factors, but one important observation is that as we age, SM gradually loses its ability to regenerate itself (particularly following resistance physical exercises). This is partly due to a reduced number of stem cells within the SM as we age. (SM stem cells are needed to make new SM fibres.) What this means is that as we age, we gradually lose the ability to repair micro-trauma to our SM fibres, and this manifests as reduced SM bulk, weakness and reduced functionality. The term 'sarcopenia' is sometimes used to define marked loss of SM mass, and it will not be a surprise for you to hear that sarcopenia is much commoner in older age, although not exclusively an affliction of the elderly.

The second vulnerability of the SM comes from chronic disease that can impact negatively on the SM through inflammatory and other hormonal signals. A weakened army is more vulnerable to attack and attrition. Any chronic illness can 'turbocharge' the normal aging process, sometimes referred to as 'secondary aging'. As we get older, we are more likely to develop chronic disease, and this can then create a double whammy for the poor SM.

The third vulnerability? Sedentariness. A stationary army is a sitting duck for attack! Sedentariness involves any activity where we sit or lie down. This is not to be recommended on a battlefield, unless playing dead that is! Most of us underestimate the negative impact of sedentariness on our SM mass and function and our metabolic health. Unfortunately, a vicious circle can ensue in which diminished SM mass reduces physical strength and limits movement, thereby promoting sedentariness that in turn further diminishes SM mass, with inevitable metabolic and thermogenic decline (1, 12). In short, sedentariness begets sedentariness, with diminished SM mass as a mediator. The answer? Avoid sedentariness like the plague, from the get-go!

The fourth vulnerability of the SM may come as a surprise. This is because it often results from our efforts to lose weight. To continue our analogy, we can use the adage, 'an army marches on its stomach'. Deprive an army of food, and they become more vulnerable to attack. The problem is that our traditional approach to weight loss, whether through caloric restriction, bariatric surgery or GLP-1 injections ('skinny jabs'), implements a 'Negative Energy Balance' (NEB), in which metabolic rate exceeds caloric intake. Over time, the body responds to NEB through 'eating' itself! Essentially, the body needs to seek an alternate fuel source, and the SM is an early port of call. Protein within the SM is broken down into its constituent amino acids which are then either oxidised or converted to glucose (sugar) within the liver through a process called 'gluconeogenesis' (13). The glucose can then be used to make ATP. Concurrently, there is down-regulation of the synthesis of protein within SM. Fat tissue is, of course, another port of call for an alternate fuel source.

During any sustained period of NEB through whatever means, only around 75% of body weight loss comes from fat tissue, the remaining 25% from lean tissues, mainly the SM (13, 14). The sad reality is that our traditional approach to weight loss through NEB results in collateral damage through loss of SM mass. In recent times, there has been much interest and concern regarding the loss of SM mass through use of GLP-1 injections ('skinny jabs') like Tirzepatide (Mounjaro) in which a new benchmark of >20% body weight loss has now been reached (15). In one study on GLP-1 therapies, 20–40% of total body weight loss came from lean tissues like SM (16). I discuss further this unfortunate side effect of these therapies later in the chapter.

Related to the adverse effects of NEB on our SM, a particularly unfavourable scenario occurs with 'yo-yo dieting', in which dietary caloric restrictions are implemented recurrently over a prolonged time, interspersed with episodes of weight regain, each cycle often lasting many months (17, 18). This is really bad news for the SM. The reason is that during weight regain following initial weight loss, a greater proportion of this is through fat tissue rather than SM (17, 19). In one study on postmenopausal women, it was shown that for every cycle of weight loss and weight regain, there is around a 10% drop in overall SM mass (17, 19). We should avoid 'yo-yo dieting'.

The fifth and final vulnerability of SM comes from obesity itself. This is apt, as obesity restricts our ability to move and can impede physical fitness. This is one reason why the British Army requires a BMI range between 18 and 28 $kg\,m^{-2}$ for all potential recruits. Indeed, reduced physical ability to move is one indirect reason why obesity can lead to diminished SM mass. However, there are also direct effects. Fat tissue and SM are usually considered as separate entities. However, they function as a single unit, an 'adipo-muscle axis' (AMA) (12). Furthermore, fat and SM are closely linked anatomically, with the former often surrounding and encasing the latter. This close anatomical proximity enables crosstalk between fat and SM, mediated primarily through hormonal signals released from each tissue in a 'paracrine' fashion (paracrine just means hormonal signals acting locally).

Fat tissue releases a plethora of hormonal signals ('adipokines') that are regulated by multiple factors (12). Many adipokines are released to a degree that is commensurate with the mass of fat tissue. Therefore, in obesity more adipokines are released and their signals become stronger. Around half of the adipokines released from fat have direct negative effects on the SM, including the suppression of SM myogenesis (formation of new SM fibres from stem cells) and SM hypertrophy (ability to 'bulk up' SM through resistance physical activity) (20). Many of these adipokines also worsen insulin sensitivity within the SM, which further impairs the metabolic function of the SM. Some adipokines can also impair the function of mitochondria within the SM. This can further limit the repair of SM fibres and their regeneration from stem cells (21). This crosstalk is not a one-way street, however. The SM is not just some mute listening post that dances to whatever music the fat tissue pumps out. Conversely, the SM is a right little chatterbox with a vocabulary of over 600 words (or 'myokines', chemicals that are released from the SM) (1, 22).

Unlike the fat-released adipokines that tend just to convey a constant moan from excessive fat tissue and create a rather negative atmosphere in the process, myokines convey a much more upbeat message from the SM and in the process create a feeling of well-being that is shared by many of us literally, after engaging in physical exercise. However, the SM only tends to become a chatty man (or chatty women) when it is contracting during physical exercise, when myokines are released from the SM. Myokines mediate beneficial effects including optimised repair and regeneration of the SM (particularly after physical exercise), down-regulation of the surrounding fat tissue, in addition to mediating improved insulin sensitivity (and therefore metabolic efficiency) and anti-inflammatory effects in both the SM and fat tissue. Think of fat tissue and the SM that it surrounds and encases as being a long-suffering married couple that are locked in an eternal embrace: 'Fred the Fat' and 'Skarlet the SM'. Fred is quite negative in his outlooks and spends all his time moaning to Skarlet about getting fatter and about her not contracting enough. In the process, poor Skarlet becomes downtrodden and diminished in her size and ability to cope. Thankfully though, Skarlet is much more positive in her outlook, and through contracting more, she creates a feeling of well-being in both her and Fred, thereby counteracting Fred's inherent negativity. If Skarlet contracts hard and long enough, she can even quell Fred's negativity completely, and happiness will prevail (*fig 4.4*). In our increasingly woke culture, the male/female roles of Fred and Skarlet can

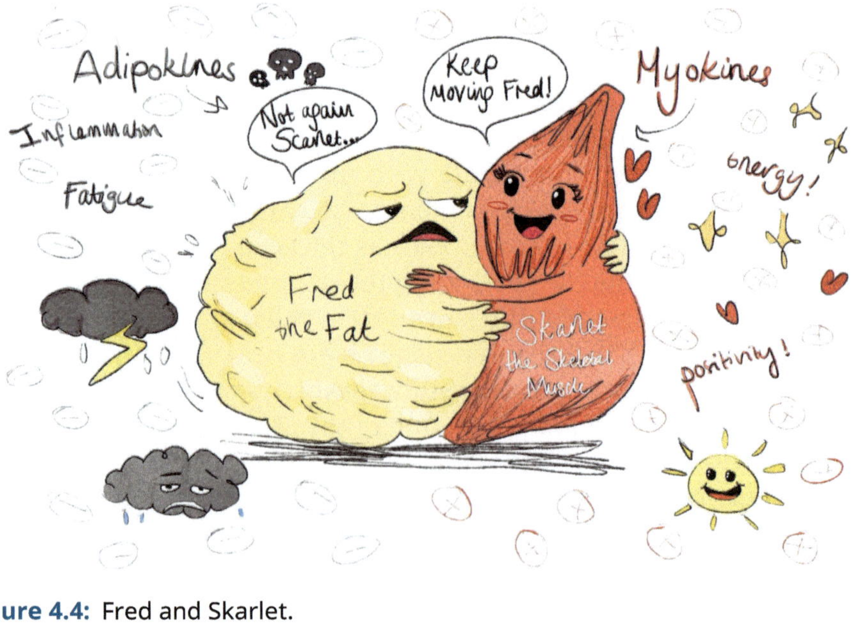

Figure 4.4: Fred and Skarlet.

be interchanged with Francesca and Sam. I think our little interlude here works better though with Fred and Skarlet, and in this spirit, I wanted to say thank goodness for women! (And I genuinely mean that.).

The Best Defence Is a Good Offence

So, what can we conclude so far? As we age, we lose SM. If we develop a chronic illness, we lose SM. If we adopt a sedentary lifestyle, we lose SM. If we try to lose weight through the traditional approach of NEB, we lose SM. If we gain weight and become obese, we lose SM.

Oh my, where on Earth do we turn to, and what can we do? Well, the clue is in the title of this subsection: we need to defend our SM by going on the offensive, which in this context means proactively striving to protect our SM as best we can.

Although maintaining our peak SM mass into older age seems like an almost impossible task, there are lifestyle strategies that we can all adopt to optimise our SM mass and function and to mitigate against and limit the inevitable decline in SM mass and function that occurs during the normal aging process. Furthermore, there are drug therapies currently in development that act directly on SM to optimise SM mass and function. Indeed, any strategy for the effective prevention and management of obesity should have at its core a clear focus on the optimisation of SM mass and function. Given the age-related demise of SM and its inherent vulnerability, we should strive to optimise our peak SM mass (achieved in our early 20s) and beyond that to limit its decline. Unfortunately, damage limitation is the name of the game for much of our adult life. In this section, I outline the main lifestyle strategies that we can adopt for protecting our SM and then discuss the role of possible future pharmacotherapies.

The main lifestyle strategy to protect our SM combines a high-protein diet (HPD) with resistance physical exercise (6). A HPD refers to any diet that has a protein intake higher than the usual recommended dietary allowance ($0.8\,g\,kg^{-1}\,day^{-1}$) (13), with the source of dietary protein being from either plants or animals (23). The 'Mediterranean diet' (consisting primarily of vegetables, fruit, cereals and olive oil) is replete with protein and has particularly favourable effects on the SM and reduces cardiovascular risk (24–26). A HPD mitigates against the loss of SM mass, including in the context of NEB induced by both caloric restriction (13, 27–29) and increased physical activity (13, 30).

So, protein in our diet is important, and this can come from both plants and animals. But proteins come in all sorts of shapes and sizes. Which begs the question, which protein is best for SM? It turns out that proteins that contain 'branched-chain amino acids' are particularly well suited to optimise SM mass through stimulated SM protein synthesis and reduced SM proteolysis (13, 31). The amino acid, leucine, is particularly favourable to the SM (13, 32). Leucine-rich foods include plants such as legumes, nuts and soybeans, meats (chicken, beef and turkey), fish (salmon and tuna) and some dairy products (yoghurt and cottage cheese). In addition, whey protein has a high leucine content and was shown to have beneficial effects on SM strength and physical performance in older adults (33).

A key learning point is that to optimise our SM mass and function, we need to adopt a HPD *concurrent* with increased resistance physical exercise (in which the SM contracts against an external force or resistance) (34). Importantly, if we adopt a HPD on its own without resistance physical exercise, this can worsen our metabolic status, contribute towards weight gain through increased fat mass and even worsen SM mass and function (35, 36). Think of it like buying some perishable food from the shop. That food is only useful to us if we then eat it within its sell-by date, otherwise it can spoil, become inedible and we then lose out. The benefit of perishable food to us is contingent on us eating it whilst still edible. Similarly, HPD is only useful if we combine it with resistance physical exercise. But why? The reason is that when we eat a load of protein, this needs to go somewhere, and if the HPD is combined with resistance physical exercise, this provides a stimulus for the uptake of amino acids from the blood into the SM to repair micro-trauma to the sarcomeres (a normal process during resistance physical exercise) (12). Without this stimulus, there is conversion of excessive dietary protein into fat (via initial conversion to glucose [sugar] through gluconeogenesis within the liver), bypassing the SM. Other forms of physical activity (aerobic and combined resistance and aerobic) also have favourable metabolic effects, including improved SM function, although resistance physical exercise appears to be particularly useful to optimise SM mass and function (21). Finally, excessive dietary protein without concurrent resistance physical exercise can also put additional strain on the kidneys (37) and stimulate the synthesis of urea (that requires additional energy and can contribute towards NEB) (38).

The rise of the GLP-1 class (with overall weight loss of >20% in the case of Tirzepatide) has brought to the fore a renewed interest in the SM and innovations to protect our SM in the context of NEB, especially with GLP-1 therapies. One area of particular interest relates to the control of SM growth and development. The SM is quite dynamic, and stem cells within the SM can produce new SM tissue under certain conditions. There are a couple of myokines called 'myostatin' and 'Activin A' that inhibit the process of producing new SM from stem cells (1, 39). There are novel therapies in development that can inhibit the action of myostatin and Activin A, thereby enabling new SM tissue to develop from SM-related stem cells (through the release of a brake on this process). 'Bimagrumab' (a 'monoclonal antibody') is one such therapy and has shown favourable effects on body composition in a 'diet-induced obese' mouse model, including reduced fat mass, increased SM mass and preservation of SM mass in the context of GLP-1-induced NEB (39). In a human-based study in participants with T2D and obesity, Bimagrumab reduced fat mass and increased lean (including SM) mass (40). In a further human-based study of community-dwelling older adults with sarcopenia and limited mobility, Bimagrumab resulted in an increase in thigh muscle volume and improved walking speed for those with a slower walking speed at baseline (41). Beyond Bimagrumab, there are other novel therapies that can also improve body composition. These include 'Azelaprag' (although no longer in active clinical development at the time of writing) that acts on the receptor for apelin (an adipokine released from fat tissue) (42, 43) and 'Monlunabant' that acts on the peripheral 'endocannabinoid' system that influences the uptake, assimilation and metabolism of nutrients following their absorption from the gut (44). This is the future of obesity management. A future in which body composition, and in particular SM mass and function are optimised. These pharmacotherapeutic innovations will have applicability in multiple clinical scenarios including to mitigate against the loss of SM mass in response to GLP-1-based therapies (and other NEB-based weight-loss strategies), and as we age with limited ability to engage in healthy lifestyle behaviours that include resistance physical exercises.

To conclude this chapter, we need to recognise that our traditional perspective of obesity is 'fat-centric'. Accordingly, our approach to the management of obesity is to reduce body weight through loosing fat tissue. As explained, the problem with this approach is that losing weight also usually results in the loss of SM mass with its associated adverse metabolic sequelae. I would argue that obesity is as much about the status of SM (mass and function) as it is about fat tissue mass. Our SMs are surrounded, encased and literally and figuratively eclipsed by fat tissue. It is time for our SMs to re-emerge from the gloominess and subordination of fat encasement and to assume a central position alongside fat tissue. It is time for us to shift our perspective towards an 'adipo-muscle ratio' (AMR), as I discussed in Chapter 3: – a perspective in which we focus on the optimisation of body composition (with reduced fat tissue mass and preserved or enhanced SM mass) rather than simply losing body weight (in which fat and SM mass are usually both reduced). This is a key challenge for the future of effective obesity management. A challenge that we all need to step up to.

References

1. Merz KE, Thurmond DC. Role of skeletal muscle in insulin resistance and glucose uptake. Compr Physiol. 2020;10(3):785–809.
2. Janssen I, Heymsfield SB, Wang ZM, Ross R. Skeletal muscle mass and distribution in 468 men and women aged 18-88 yr. J Appl Physiol (1985). 2000;89(1):81–8.
3. Li H, Wang C, Li L, Li L. Skeletal muscle non-shivering thermogenesis as an attractive strategy to combat obesity. Life Sci. 2021;269:119024.
4. Tomiya S, Tamura Y, Kouzaki K, Kotani T, Wakabayashi Y, Noda M, et al. Cast immobilization of hindlimb upregulates sarcolipin expression in atrophied skeletal muscles and increases thermogenesis in C57BL/6J mice. Am J Physiol Regul Integr Comp Physiol. 2019;317(5):R649–R61.
5. DeFronzo RA, Tripathy D. Skeletal muscle insulin resistance is the primary defect in type 2 diabetes. Diabetes Care. 2009;32(Suppl 2):S157–63.
6. Argiles JM, Campos N, Lopez-Pedrosa JM, Rueda R, Rodriguez-Manas L. Skeletal muscle regulates metabolism via interorgan crosstalk: roles in health and disease. J Am Med Dir Assoc. 2016;17(9):789–96.
7. Taylor AH, Doust J, Webborn N. Randomised controlled trial to examine the effects of a GP exercise referral programme in Hailsham, East Sussex, on modifiable coronary heart disease risk factors. J Epidemiol Community Health. 1998;52(9):595–601.
8. Rodriguez-Rodero S, Fernandez-Morera JL, Menendez-Torre E, Calvanese V, Fernandez AF, Fraga MF. Aging genetics and aging. Aging Dis. 2011;2(3):186–95.
9. Shen X, Wang C, Zhou X, Zhou W, Hornburg D, Wu S, et al. Nonlinear dynamics of multi-omics profiles during human aging. Nat Aging. 2024;4(11):1619–34.
10. Reyes-Farias M, Fos-Domenech J, Serra D, Herrero L, Sanchez-Infantes D. White adipose tissue dysfunction in obesity and aging. Biochem Pharmacol. 2021;192:114723.
11. Kedlian VR, Wang Y, Liu T, Chen X, Bolt L, Tudor C, et al. Human skeletal muscle aging atlas. Nat Aging. 2024;4(5):727–44.
12. Barber TM, Kabisch S, Pfeiffer AFH, Weickert MO. Optimised skeletal muscle mass as a key strategy for obesity management. Metabolites. 2025;15(2):85.
13. Carbone JW, McClung JP, Pasiakos SM. Skeletal muscle responses to negative energy balance: effects of dietary protein. Adv Nutr. 2012;3(2):119–26.
14. Weinheimer EM, Sands LP, Campbell WW. A systematic review of the separate and combined effects of energy restriction and exercise on fat-free mass in middle-aged and older adults: implications for sarcopenic obesity. Nutr Rev. 2010;68(7):375–88.
15. Aronne LJ, Sattar N, Horn DB, Bays HE, Wharton S, Lin WY, et al. Continued treatment with tirzepatide for maintenance of weight reduction in adults with obesity: the SURMOUNT-4 randomized clinical trial. JAMA. 2024;331(1):38–48.
16. Dubin RL, Heymsfield SB, Ravussin E, Greenway FL. Glucagon-like peptide-1 receptor agonist-based agents and weight loss composition: filling the gaps. Diabetes Obes Metab. 2024;26(12):5503–18.

17. Weickert MO. Nutritional modulation of insulin resistance. Scientifica (Cairo). 2012;2012:424780.
18. Pi-Sunyer FX. Weight loss in type 2 diabetic patients. Diabetes Care. 2005;28(6):1526–7.
19. Beavers KM, Lyles MF, Davis CC, Wang X, Beavers DP, Nicklas BJ. Is lost lean mass from intentional weight loss recovered during weight regain in postmenopausal women? Am J Clin Nutr. 2011;94(3):767–74.
20. Collins KH, Gui C, Ely EV, Lenz KL, Harris CA, Guilak F, et al. Leptin mediates the regulation of muscle mass and strength by adipose tissue. J Physiol. 2022;600(16):3795–817.
21. Axelrod CL, Dantas WS, Kirwan JP. Sarcopenic obesity: emerging mechanisms and therapeutic potential. Metabolism. 2023;146:155639.
22. Kirk B, Feehan J, Lombardi G, Duque G. Muscle, bone, and fat crosstalk: the biological role of myokines, osteokines, and adipokines. Curr Osteoporos Rep. 2020;18(4):388–400.
23. Markova M, Pivovarova O, Hornemann S, Sucher S, Frahnow T, Wegner K, et al. Isocaloric diets high in animal or plant protein reduce liver fat and inflammation in individuals with type 2 diabetes. Gastroenterology. 2017;152(3):571–85 e8.
24. Barber TM, Kabisch S, Pfeiffer AFH, Weickert MO. The effects of the mediterranean diet on health and gut microbiota. Nutrients. 2023;15(9):2150.
25. Konieczna J, Ruiz-Canela M, Galmes-Panades AM, Abete I, Babio N, Fiol M, et al. An energy-reduced mediterranean diet, physical activity, and body composition: an interim subgroup analysis of the PREDIMED-plus randomized clinical trial. JAMA Netw Open. 2023;6(10):e2337994.
26. Di Rosa C, Lattanzi G, Spiezia C, Imperia E, Piccirilli S, Beato I, et al. Mediterranean diet versus very low-calorie ketogenic diet: effects of reaching 5% body weight loss on body composition in subjects with overweight and with obesity-a cohort study. Int J Environ Res Public Health. 2022;19(20):13040.
27. Gordon MM, Bopp MJ, Easter L, Miller GD, Lyles MF, Houston DK, et al. Effects of dietary protein on the composition of weight loss in postmenopausal women. J Nutr Health Aging. 2008;12(8):505–9.
28. Farnsworth E, Luscombe ND, Noakes M, Wittert G, Argyiou E, Clifton PM. Effect of a high-protein, energy-restricted diet on body composition, glycemic control, and lipid concentrations in overweight and obese hyperinsulinemic men and women. Am J Clin Nutr. 2003;78(1):31–9.
29. Skov AR, Toubro S, Ronn B, Holm L, Astrup A. Randomized trial on protein vs carbohydrate in ad libitum fat reduced diet for the treatment of obesity. Int J Obes Relat Metab Disord. 1999;23(5):528–36.
30. Pikosky MA, Smith TJ, Grediagin A, Castaneda-Sceppa C, Byerley L, Glickman EL, et al. Increased protein maintains nitrogen balance during exercise-induced energy deficit. Med Sci Sports Exerc. 2008;40(3):505–12.
31. Layman DK. Protein quantity and quality at levels above the RDA improves adult weight loss. J Am Coll Nutr. 2004;23(6 Suppl):631S–6S.
32. Pasiakos SM, McClung HL, McClung JP, Margolis LM, Andersen NE, Cloutier GJ, et al. Leucine-enriched essential amino acid supplementation during moderate steady state exercise enhances postexercise muscle protein synthesis. Am J Clin Nutr. 2011;94(3):809–18.

33. Al-Rawhani AH, Adznam SN, Abu Zaid Z, Md Yusop NB, M Sallehuddin H, Alshawsh MA. Effectiveness of whey protein supplementation on muscle strength and physical performance of older adults: a systematic review and meta-analysis of randomized clinical trials. Clin Nutr. 2024;43(10):2412–26.
34. Morton RW, Murphy KT, McKellar SR, Schoenfeld BJ, Henselmans M, Helms E, et al. A systematic review, meta-analysis and meta-regression of the effect of protein supplementation on resistance training-induced gains in muscle mass and strength in healthy adults. Br J Sports Med. 2018;52(6):376–84.
35. Weickert MO, Roden M, Isken F, Hoffmann D, Nowotny P, Osterhoff M, et al. Effects of supplemented isoenergetic diets differing in cereal fiber and protein content on insulin sensitivity in overweight humans. Am J Clin Nutr. 2011;94(2):459–71.
36. Weickert MO, Pfeiffer AF. Signalling mechanisms linking hepatic glucose and lipid metabolism. Diabetologia. 2006;49(8):1732–41.
37. Verreijen AM, Engberink MF, Memelink RG, van der Plas SE, Visser M, Weijs PJ. Effect of a high protein diet and/or resistance exercise on the preservation of fat free mass during weight loss in overweight and obese older adults: a randomized controlled trial. Nutr J. 2017;16(1):10.
38. Madiraju AK, Alves T, Zhao X, Cline GW, Zhang D, Bhanot S, et al. Argininosuccinate synthetase regulates hepatic AMPK linking protein catabolism and ureagenesis to hepatic lipid metabolism. Proc Natl Acad Sci U S A. 2016;113(24):E3423–30.
39. Nunn E, Jaiswal N, Gavin M, Uehara K, Stefkovich M, Drareni K, et al. Antibody blockade of activin type II receptors preserves skeletal muscle mass and enhances fat loss during GLP-1 receptor agonism. Mol Metab. 2024;80:101880.
40. Heymsfield SB, Coleman LA, Miller R, Rooks DS, Laurent D, Petricoul O, et al. Effect of bimagrumab vs placebo on body fat mass among adults with type 2 diabetes and obesity: a phase 2 randomized clinical trial. JAMA Netw Open. 2021;4(1):e2033457.
41. Rooks D, Praestgaard J, Hariry S, Laurent D, Petricoul O, Perry RG, et al. Treatment of sarcopenia with bimagrumab: results from a phase II, randomized, controlled, proof-of-concept study. J Am Geriatr Soc. 2017;65(9):1988–95.
42. Trivedi A, Mather O, Vega S, Hutton S, Hellawell J, Lee E. A phase I, open-label, single-dose study to evaluate the pharmacokinetics, safety, and tolerability of AMG 986 in healthy Japanese subjects. Drugs R D. 2022;22(2):141–6.
43. Chapman FA, Maguire JJ, Newby DE, Davenport AP, Dhaun N. Targeting the apelin system for the treatment of cardiovascular diseases. Cardiovasc Res. 2023;119(17):2683–96.
44. Crater GD, Lalonde K, Ravenelle F, Harvey M, Despres JP. Effects of CB1R inverse agonist, INV-202, in patients with features of metabolic syndrome. A randomized, placebo-controlled, double-blind phase 1b study. Diabetes Obes Metab. 2024;26(2):642–9.

5 The Gut Microbiota

Imagine living in your poo! I don't think it would get great reviews on 'Tripadvisor', and moving house would be a bit of a challenge. I mean, no amount of polishing would enable you to square that circle! Disgusting as this little thought experiment is, your poo is home to countless trillions of microbes who call it home. And not just any old home for that matter. To a microbe, your poo is luxury, all-inclusive, 5-star accommodation. More specifically, the inside of your large bowel (colon) is where all the action happens, and your microbiota basks in a glorious environment, protected from the outside world and with a plentiful supply of nutrients. The lack of a sea view and the overpowering stench might be something to complain about, but hey, who cares about the view and the smell when you don't have eyes or a nose?! Protection, nutrients and the ability to replicate are all that really matter to a microbe. The act of defecation is where it all goes a bit Pete Tong for the poor little microbe that lives in your poo, and I guess at that point it is time for it to say 'goodbye' to your colon from whence it came and 'hello' to a whole new and exciting life in the sewers.

The microbes that live in your poo and in your gut are the 'gut microbiota', the focus for this chapter. 'Microbiota' is an umbrella term that includes bacteria and other forms of microbe such as viruses, fungi, amoebozoa and archaea (1, 2). Your microbiota extends well beyond your gut and includes any surface exposed to the outside environment. This includes your skin, genitourinary tract and respiratory tract. However, 70% of your microbiota resides in your colon (3). This is around 100 trillion microbes (4), about the same as the number of stars in the observable universe. Imagine that: a universe of microbes contained within your colon! In fact, the number of microbes living in your colon outnumber your own cells. In a real sense, you are more microbe than human. Hang on a minute though, I hear you say. How can the weight of your poo compete with the weight of your body for cell number? (The weight of the contents of your gut is around 2 kg.) Well, the reason is that your microbes are much smaller than your own cells, and therefore more of them can pack into a colon-sized space. This is especially the case for viruses which are around 100–1,000 times smaller than human cells.

Bacteria and microbes receive a bad press. There are whole industries that have evolved to eradicate them, with antibacterial sprays, disinfectants and antibiotics, all designed to kill bacteria and other microbes to protect us. We tend to think of bacteria as being harmful and something to avoid at all costs. This anti-bacteria mindset is hardly surprising when one considers that historically, infectious disease was a major threat to human life, and indeed still is in parts of the world, with around 600,000 people dying from malaria each year globally. It is ironic therefore that bacteria and microbes are also essential for our survival, to a degree that you may find surprising. Although the media are catching up with our recent insights into the health benefits of bacteria and other microbes, they also tend to dichotomise this topic, as they often do for medical-related topics in general. For example, you will sometimes hear media speak about 'good' and 'bad' bacteria. Doubtless this is sometimes the case. The bacterium that causes plague, for example, *Yersinia pestis*, is presumably always going to be bad, and we should avoid it like, well, the plague! However, for other forms of bacteria, we should probably avoid the attribution of a 'good' or 'bad' status; otherwise we will get ourselves into a bit of a pickle. For example, some forms of bacteria like certain strains of *E. coli* can cause serious illness; other strains of the same bacterium are harmless to us, and yet other strains of *E. coli* (forming part of our gut microbiota) are even beneficial to us. The bacterium, *Neisseria meningitidis*, is responsible for the most severe form of meningitis (septicaemia) and yet forms part of our microbiota, residing on the mucosal surfaces of the throat and nose in around 10% of us (carriers) without seemingly causing any harm or illness (neither 'good' nor 'bad', just 'there'). Whilst harmless most of the time, this bacterium can also cause fatal septicaemia. We do not fully understand what factors influence the pathogenicity of this bacterium in each of us and ultimately what determines who gets ill and who doesn't.

Our universe of gut microbiota helps us to survive. We co-evolved with our gut microbiota over unimaginable timescales, hundreds of millions of years in fact. Our immune systems have learned to tolerate our gut microbiota, which is a good thing when you think about it. But more than that, our immune system depends on our gut microbiota for its normal development. Think of your gut microbiota as a training ground for an army (your immune system), equipped with assault courses, mock-up fighting environments and rifle practice. Just as rigorous training strengthens and prepares an army, so too your own immune system

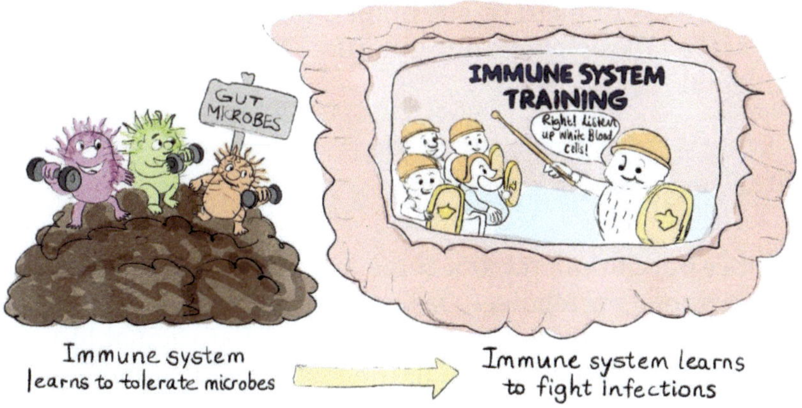

Figure 5.1: The poo-based training ground.

relies upon your gut microbiota for its training. In this way, you can see that there is an interdependence between your gut microbiota and immune system, the former training the latter and the latter tolerating the former – a truly symbiotic relationship. In fact, one could even consider the gut microbiota and immune system as a single integrated unit rather than as separate entities (*fig 5.1*).

During this century, there has been a renaissance in our understanding of the role of gut microbiota in health and disease. The gut microbiota plays a key role in health and well-being and in the development of much 21st century chronic ill health, including autoimmune conditions (when the immune system attacks part of your own body), food intolerances, atopies (allergic conditions like asthma, hay fever and eczema), chronic inflammatory and neuro-psychiatric conditions (5). Indeed, the gut microbiota also plays a role in the development of mental health conditions like depression and anxiety. And yes, you have guessed it, the gut microbiota also influences our predisposition to the development of obesity and other obesity-related dysmetabolic conditions, through their effects on our appetite, metabolism, body weight and composition. That is the reason I have devoted a whole chapter to its discussion. I will divide this discussion into three main parts. The first is to consider the origins and provenance of the gut microbiota. Where does it come from? In the second part, I will reveal the fascinating conversations that occur between our gut microbiota and brain: it turns out that they are chattering away to each other all the time, and they each have a lot to say to one another! Finally, I will discuss strategies to optimise our gut microbiota to promote a future full of health and well-being. For this, we need to take ownership and shift our perspective of our gut microbiota from alien to that of organ status, essential for our health and well-being, requiring protection and nurture just like our heart or any other organ. In this spirit, we should probably stop talking about our gut microbiota as 'them' and instead as an integral part of 'us'.

The Origins of the Gut Microbiota

Where does our gut microbiota come from? When we are newly born, our gut microbiota is relatively restricted. The initial seeding of our gut microbiota depends on our mode of delivery. For vaginal births, there is oral exposure of the newborn to the maternal microbiota, including microbiota that resides in the vagina, on the skin and, you guessed it, in the maternal gut. Studies have revealed that compared with caesarean section (C-section), neonates born vaginally develop a greater diversity and improved colonisation of their gut microbiota (6). Furthermore, compared with vaginal delivery, C-section birth can lead to long-term health problems including obesity and chronic inflammatory conditions that can extend into adulthood (6). Although these data only reveal association and there are confounders, they are nonetheless consistent with a protective effect of seeding of the newborn gut with maternally derived microbes during vaginal delivery (6).

So, the first answer to the origins of our gut microbiota is that, at least for those of us who were born vaginally, our mother's own microbiota (including her gut microbiota) helps us to establish our own gut microbiota at birth. The story doesn't end there though. During the early part of the 21st century, our understanding of the constituents of human breast milk was transformed. Although once thought of as sterile, it turns out that human breast milk contains an abundance of diverse microbes that play a key role in the colonisation and establishment of the infant gut microbiota (6). These microbes are anaerobes and the type found in the gut microbiota. The implication is that there is a mechanism in the lactating mother, in which there is translocation of her own gut microbiota across her gut wall, and somehow these microbes are then transported into her breast milk for her suckling infant. Now isn't that just an incredible thought? The physiology of this 'entero-mammary pathway', what controls it and how it works are incompletely understood and areas of ongoing research. But we know it must exist, and we can surmise that evolution has endowed our species with a rather cool way of turbo-charging the infant gut microbiota, through seeding from the mother's own gut microbiota via her breast milk. Furthermore, although our gut microbiota is modifiable through lifestyle changes, as outlined later in this chapter, it turns out that our maternally-derived gut microbiota that we acquire at birth and during infancy has a degree of permanence and is more resistant to change. This then is one of the many ways in which our mothers stay close to us, even as adults, through a shared gut microbiota.

Listening in on Conversations Between the Gut Microbiota and Brain

Intuitively, we know that there is a close connection between our brain and gut. It is written into our language with colloquialisms such as 'butterflies in the tummy', 'sick to the stomach' and 'gut feeling'. The origins of our language and expressions can tell us a lot about our biology and physiology. It is not coincidental that these gut-related expressions exist and often inform us about how we feel about something. This includes mentally comparing 'gut-feelings' about counterfactual future scenarios, that in turn helps us to make decisions. It is also no coincidence that mental health problems often coexist with disorders (including dysfunction) of the gastrointestinal tract.

The close links between the gut and the brain should not really surprise us when we consider the intricate ways in which the gut and brain are linked: the so-called 'gut-brain axis'. For this to be revealed in its full glory, I would like to invite you to become imaginary members of the 'Government Communications Headquarters' (better known simply as 'GCHQ'), the United Kingdom's main listening post. Instead of listening in to conversations between spies though, we will be listening in to conversations between the gut (and by implication the gut microbiota) and the brain. The first interception point from where we can listen is the main 'wired' link between the gut and the brain, the 'vagus nerve'. Of all nerves, I think the vagus is one of my favourites. In case you were wondering, it is not named after Johnny or after that city in Nevada, well known for its gambling and 'drive-through' weddings! Rather, it has the same origin as the word, 'vagrant', and in Latin means 'wandering' (not the pondering type of wondering, but the type where you go for a wander round a city, for example). Just like a vagrant who wanders idly from place to place, so too the vagus nerve takes its wandering course. What a brilliant analogy! Unlike many nerves that take the most direct route to wherever they are destined (analogous to a 'geodesic' long-haul flight path across the globe), the vagus nerve wanders about all over the place, taking in all the scenery as it goes on its merry way. It is a remarkably curious nerve! The vagus nerve starts its wandering course in the brainstem and has connections with organs and peripheral tissues throughout the body, including extensive and intricate innervations throughout the gut. In fact, the gut is one of the most highly innervated systems in the body, thanks to the course of the vagus nerve (*fig 5.2*).

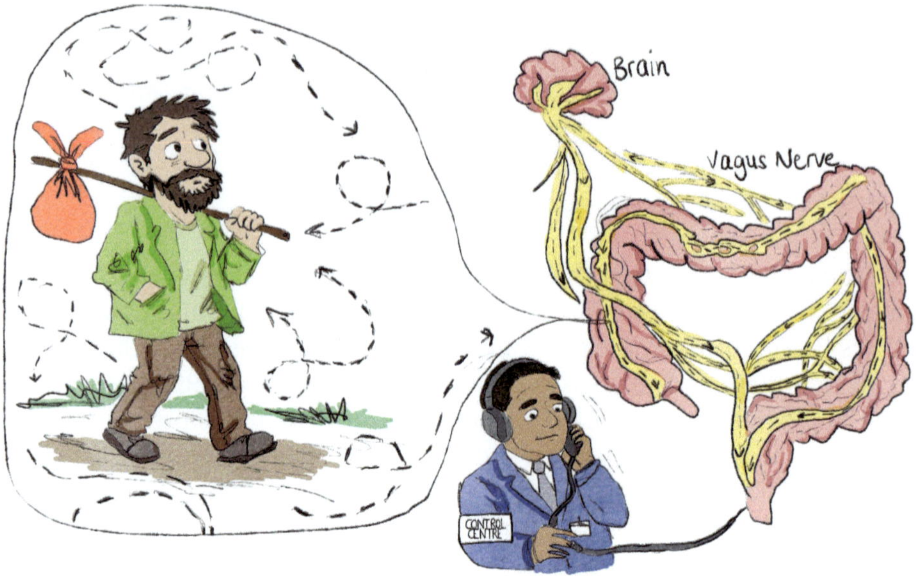

Figure 5.2: The vagus nerve as it wanders like a vagrant.

Importantly for our discussion, the vagus nerve facilitates a two-way communication stream between the gut microbiota and the brain. The signals coming from the brain are part of the 'autonomic' (or automatic) nervous system and carry 'parasympathetic' signals. These signals are not under our conscious control and predominate when we are in a relaxed state, like when we are sleeping, for example. Think of these signals as being the opposite of the adrenaline-charged 'fight or flight' response that occurs when you experience stress (mediated by the separate 'sympathetic' nervous system). The parasympathetic signals that travel from the brain down the vagus nerve have a calming effect on the body, and I think this makes the vagus a particularly cool nerve. In short, it is the vagus nerve (along with our highly developed frontal cortices) that helps us to avoid being chimp-like in our behaviour, allowing us to 'calm down, calm down' (that works best if pronounced in a Scouser accent!). These vagal parasympathetic signals also influence the function of the gut, facilitating digestion and assimilation of nutrients and optimising the function of our gut microbiota. Sensory signals from the gut (and other organs and tissues innervated by the vagus nerve) travel in the opposite direction, from the gut to the brain. These 'afferent' nerve signals alert the brain to any inflammation within the peripheral organs (through pain signals) and indeed immerse the brain with signals that influence the physical feelings of emotion that are familiar to most of us. These include love, 'heartbreak', 'heart sink', 'joy in my heart' and the gut-related feelings alluded to earlier.

How do we know that the vagus nerve is used by the gut microbiota to communicate with the brain and vice versa? It is important at this stage to highlight that much of our understanding of the gut microbiota, and its role in obesity and other aspects of health and disease stem from studies in rodents. There are some human studies, but relatively few and detailed experiments are obviously much easier to perform in rodents than in humans. Data from one rodent-based study particularly is relevant for our discussion. In this study, it was shown that mice fed with a strain of lactobacillus (a type of gut microbe) over a prolonged period resulted in changes in the expression of certain neurotransmitters in the brain, changes in behaviour (specifically reduced anxiety- and depression-related behaviours) and reductions in the stress hormone, cortisol. When the same experiment was repeated in vagotomised mice (where the vagus nerve is severed and therefore ceases to function), the effects outlined above did not occur (7). This experiment provides proof of concept that the gut microbiota influence brain function and behaviour, albeit in a rodent model, via signalling within the vagus nerve. In addition to direct links between the gut and the brain, it is likely that some of the vagal signals between the gut and the brain travel via (and are mediated by) the liver (8).

Data from other rodent-based studies reveal that gut microbiota influences the expression of multiple neurotransmitters and neuroreceptors and accordingly also influence emotionally driven behaviours. This includes the 'Gamma-Amino Butyric Acid' (GABA) receptor, mediating the brain's main inhibitory neurotransmitter system, acting like a brake mechanism, essential for the normal regulation of psychological and physiological processes, and implicated in the pathogenesis of anxiety and depression (7). The gut microbiota also influences the brain's expression of serotonin that plays a central role in the regulation of mood and sleep. Finally, the gut microbiota influences the brain's expression of a protein called 'brain-derived neurotrophic factor' (BDNF) that is important for the development, survival and function of neurones in the brain. Rodents with a healthy gut microbiota have increased brain expression of BDNF (9), whereas rodents that were reared germ-free (and therefore have an impoverished and unhealthy gut microbiota) have diminished levels of BDNF in the brain, particularly in the hippocampus, an area of the brain that is important for memory formation, for spatial navigation and for the regulation of emotions and survival behaviours (10). It turns out that being reared germ-free also results in overactivity of the stress-hormone axis (cortisol) and increased anxiety-like behaviour (11, 12). Given that parasympathetic drive predominates in a relaxed state, free from stress and anxiety, it follows that a 'golden circuit' ensues, in which healthy and diverse gut microbiota reduce stress and anxiety, that in turn enables a predominance of parasympathetic outputs within the vagus nerve, that in turn optimises functioning of the gut, nutrient handling and nurture of the gut microbiota, that in turn...

In contrast to signalling via the vagus nerve, our second GCHQ-like interception point is the 'metabolic by-products' of the gut microbiota, the chemicals that are produced by the gut microbiota during the process of their metabolism of the nutrients that we eat. You might think that these chemical by-products are insignificant and are just eliminated from the body, but you would be wrong. It turns out that these metabolic by-products have all kinds of effects on brain function, including the control of appetite and metabolism. These chemical by-products can be absorbed into the blood across the gut wall, and whilst transitioning the gut wall they can modify the release of 'incretin' hormones that then influence the control of appetite and metabolism. These chemicals can also travel in the blood and have direct effects on brain function. (Incidentally, afferent signals within the vagus nerve from the gut to the brain likely also originate from the effects of gut microbiota-derived chemical by-products interacting with vagal nerve endings within the gut wall, as they transition through the gut wall.) One of the chemical by-products of gut microbiota metabolism that have received much attention are 'Short Chain Fatty Acids' (SCFAs) (7, 13). These are produced by a genus of bacteria within the gut called *Enterococcus* during the fermentation of dietary fibre. It has been shown that levels of *Enterococcus* in the gut and levels of SCFAs in the blood both associate with inhibitory effects on appetite control and impact positively on the control of metabolism (14). Human-based studies also reveal health benefits of SCFAs. In one study, ingested propionate (a form of SCFA) resulted in weight loss, improved insulin sensitivity and an earlier release of incretin hormones during a meal that suppressed appetite and reduced caloric intake (15).

All this GCHQ-type listening is quite tiring is it not? There is just one more final interception point and that is the gut wall itself and its mucus lining. As outlined earlier, our gut microbiota and immune systems are closely linked, and the gut and brain communicate with each other closely. Importantly though, these communication streams occur normally across a physical barrier that prevents the gut microbiota from entering the bloodstream. This physical barrier depends on both an intact gut wall and a healthy mucus lining of the gut wall. A further important factor is a high-fibre diet (the focus of Chapter 8), that provides a medium for which our gut microbiota can happily 'munch' away on. When happiness prevails in our gut microbiota, they stay well behaved and promote our health and well-being. There is a medical term for this state: eubiosis. This simply means a healthy, diverse and well-balanced gut microbiota, with all their needs provided for. In this scenario, all the stars are aligned to protect our gut wall lining, with happy microbiota munching on our dietary fibre, kept well away from an intact gut wall by a thick layer of mucus. Conversely, when unhappiness prevails and there is an imbalance within our gut microbiota, often through poor lifestyle choices, the opposite occurs. This is termed 'dysbiosis', a prerequisite of which is impoverishment of dietary fibre, with a consequent lack of a fibre medium for our gut microbiota to munch on. This means that our gut microbiota cannot thrive and instead becomes diminished in both its diversity and extent. With a lack of dietary fibre, the remaining unhappy and imbalanced gut microbiota munch away at the mucus lining of our gut instead, impairing its integrity and getting ever closer to the gut wall. Eventually, the mucus lining of the gut wall is breached, and the gut microbiota can then stimulate an inflammatory reaction within the gut wall, termed 'colitis'. Another feature of dysbiosis is that the gut wall itself (the integrity of the connections between the cells forming the gut wall) becomes less tight and more 'leaky'. In this scenario, components of the gut microbiota can leak across the gut wall and into the blood and then provoke a low-level inflammatory response in peripheral tissues that is bad for metabolic health, and negative effects on brain health that include changes in cognition, mood, neuroinflammation and neurodegeneration. This is termed 'endotoxaemia'. Many modern-day 21st century chronic illnesses are linked with dysbiosis (*fig 5.3*).

Eubiosis and dysbiosis are descriptive terms that represent two ends of a spectrum of gut health, happiness and diversity. In the last section, we need to leave our listening post at GCHQ in Cheltenham and travel along the A40, past Clarkson's pub and beyond all the way to the Ministry of Defence in London to learn not so much about how our immune system can defend us against our gut microbiota, but rather how we can defend and nurture our gut microbiota through healthy lifestyle choices, to establish and maintain eubiosis, to protect us from the development of dysbiosis and in the process to optimise our future health and well-being.

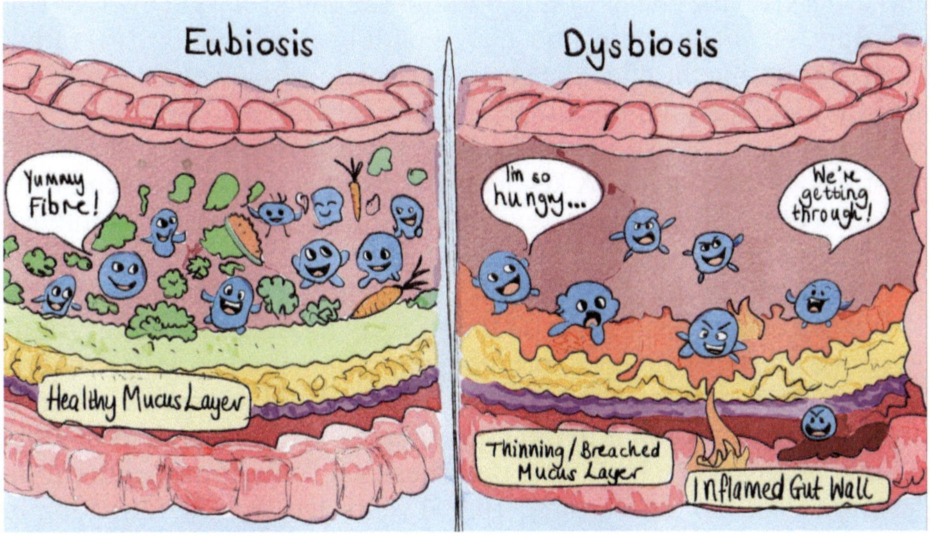

Figure 5.3: Feeding your gut microbiota.

Strategies to Optimise Our Gut Microbiota to Promote Our Health and Well-Being

Many of us are familiar with the idea of promoting our heart health or protecting and developing our brains to reduce our chance of developing ischaemic heart disease and dementia, respectively, in the future. Our notion of an organ like the heart or brain is redolent of a collection of cells that are highly organised and which perform some vital function. Unsurprisingly perhaps, up until quite recently, the idea of promoting our gut microbiota was an alien concept. Our gut microbiota doesn't really fit neatly into our traditional idea of an organ. For a start, it is composed of cells that are alien to us, which reside outside of the body (think of the body as doughnut-shaped, with a continuous hole from mouth to anus: this hole is occupied largely by the gut microbiota). Furthermore, the gut microbiota is hardly ordered but rather represents a seething mass of microbes. From the perspective of physiological function though, the gut microbiota plays as important a role as any other organ. For that reason, I think we should elevate its deserved status to that of organ.

It is worth reiterating that most of our insights in the 21st century on the impact of the gut microbiota on health and disease stem from rodent-based studies, with relatively few human-based studies. It could be said that the gut microbiota field is in its infancy, and doubtless our knowledge and insights will continue to grow in the future. As an illustration of how little we know, of the 100 trillion microbes that reside in the human colon, we have only identified around 1,000 species (3). Within the gut microbiota, there are four major microbial phyla that comprise >90% of the bacteria: *Bacteroides*, *Firmicutes*, *Actinobacteria* and *Proteobacteria* (16). Furthermore, most of the literature in this field has focused on the effects of single strains (or phyla) of a gut microbe (for example, *Firmicutes* being associated with health benefits (16)) rather than considering the effects of clusters of microbes or even the entire gut microbiota. That said, we can glean some general insights, from which we can recommend strategies for how to optimise our gut microbiota, the topic of this section. A key learning point is that when it comes to gut microbiota, diversity is key. We should all be striving to establish and maintain a diverse gut microbiota: a colonic milieu that enables a diverse variety of microbes to multiply and flourish, a state of eubiosis.

It will not come as a surprise that dietary modification forms a cornerstone lifestyle strategy to promote our gut microbiota. A fascinating archaeological study on teeth from our hominid ancestors revealed significant modifications in their gut microbiota during periods of rapid dietary change (17), including the transition from hunter-gatherer to farming Neolithic eras around 10,000 years ago and the transition to the industrialized era around 200 years ago (17). Each of these revolutions resulted in a change in our diet, including increased carbohydrate intake. More recently, in Western countries, we have adopted intake of ultra-processed foods (UPFs), which are depleted of fibre, laden with carbohydrate and fats and highly sterilised. This is really bad news from the perspective of the gut microbiota. Due to our obsession with avoiding disease from infections, we tend to live in highly sterilised environments, which further compounds our lack of exposure to microbes that could otherwise replenish our gut microbiota. It has been shown that bacteria in common fermented foods from plant and animal origins (including cheese and cured meats) reach the gut (18). This insight forms a rationale for the addition of foreign microbes into our food, in addition to a diet that includes fermentable foods like cheese, sauerkraut, kefir and kimchi, to provide continuous replenishment of our gut microbiota. In short, we and our gut microbiota co-evolved from the ingestion of lots of microbes in the food that we eat, from a tuber dug up from the ground, from a fruit plucked from a tree and from meat ripped from the skeletal remains of the latest kill (that may have been stored unrefrigerated for a few days).

Of all the macronutrients in our diet that establishes and maintains a diverse and healthy gut microbiota, dietary fibre reigns supreme (discussed in detail in Chapter 8). Plant-based foods contain dietary fibre, and we should eat a wide variety of plants in our diet. Dietary fibre provides us with multiple health benefits (19). Unfortunately, our Western diets are depleted of dietary fibre, and most of us need to increase intake of dietary fibre by around 50% (19). Dietary fibre provides a milieu, in which our gut microbiota can grow and flourish and encourages the growth of *Bifidobacteria* species that have favourable effects on health. Furthermore, *Bifidobacteria* improve the barrier function of the gut wall, thereby protecting us from any potentially harmful effects of our gut microbiota including colitis or endotoxaemia (20). Finally, dietary fibre encourages the growth of strains like *Bacteroides* and *Eubacterium* that release nutrients like folic acid and biotin that are then absorbed and utilised by us and by our gut microbiota (21).

So much for dietary fibre. What about dietary fats? For this discussion, it is important to consider each subtype of fat. The ingestion of Monounsaturated Fatty Acids (MUFAs) and Polyunsaturated Fatty Acids (PUFAs, including omega-6 and omega-3) have favourable effects on our gut microbiota. This includes foods like oily fish. However, other types of fats contain saturated fatty acids and trans-fatty acids that are typically contained in UPFs. These types of fats are bad for our gut microbiota and promote dysbiosis, low-grade inflammation within the gut wall (colitis), and leakiness of the gut wall. These unhealthy fats also encourage the growth of microbes that promote endotoxaemia and a type of bacterium called *Bilophila wadsworthia* (18) that produces hydrogen sulfide that in turn can contribute to colitis.

To summarise, eat a wide variety of plants every day. Meat, poultry and oily fish are fine, but cook them yourself from their raw states. Avoid UPFs as these deliver a double whammy to our gut microbiota, being impoverished of dietary fibre, and replete with the harmful forms of dietary fat (22). If you apply this simple mantra to your daily diet, you will be nurturing your gut microbiota. So much for diet, what about other aspects of lifestyle? There is a wealth of evidence in the medical literature on this topic, so here I will only provide a summary. In essence though, excessive alcohol is bad for our gut microbiota for two main reasons. Firstly, alcohol itself is toxic to microbes, and so results in an impoverished gut microbiota in which dysbiosis, colitis and endotoxaemia prevail. Secondly, there is an association between alcohol excess and impaired diet in which nutrient deficiencies can occur. Therefore, avoid excessive alcohol. Stress too is damaging to our gut microbiota. There are likely multiple mechanisms, but remember that being stressed often results in sympathetic overdrive in which the body and mind are in a chronically 'revved-up' state, and there is little chance for our old friend, the vagus nerve, to work its magic and deliver a calming (parasympathetic) effect on the body and gut that in turn helps our gut microbiota to flourish. Avoid sedentariness. When we engage in physical activity, our skeletal muscles release chemicals called myokines that have all kinds of favourable effects on our body, including in the gut. Our gut microbiota benefits from us being physically active. Finally, and this one will blow your mind, our gut microbiota even likes to sleep when we do. Like us, and like pretty much every cell in our body, it turns out that our gut microbiota also has a circadian or sleep-wake cycle, which is entrained to our own. Furthermore, there is evidence to suggest that if we disturb the sleep-wake cycle of our gut microbiota, this can be harmful for our metabolic health (1). Just like most of us are grouchy if woken up in the middle of the night, it turns out that the same can be said for our gut microbiota! Therefore, get good amounts of restful sleep each night and try to maintain a regular sleep-wake cycle with constant and regular sleeping and waking times, wherever possible (*fig 5.4*).

Beyond lifestyle strategies, are there any other things we can do to optimise our gut microbiota? There are probiotics that claim to have all kinds of health benefits, but I think we lack the scientific evidence currently to advocate their widespread use. Furthermore, probiotics are not usually recommended as a therapeutic option on the NHS. We do not yet have a 'crapsule' as a means of delivering gut microbiota to our colon. Currently within the NHS, faecal transplantation is only indicated for the management of patients with intractable colonic colonisation with *Clostridium difficile* (23). However, despite our understandable aversion

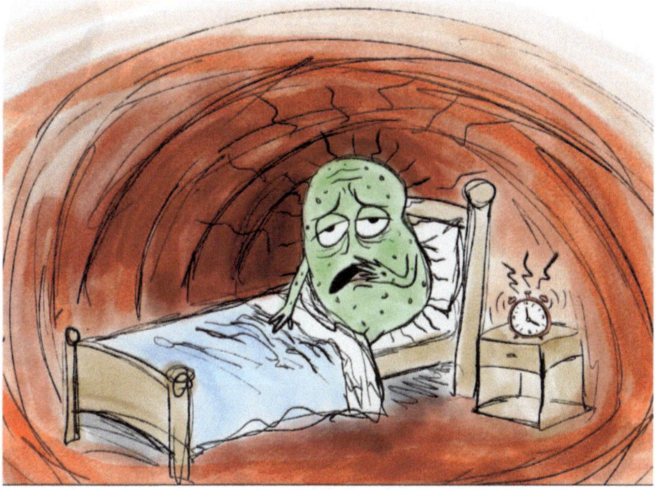

Figure 5.4: Our gut microbiota needs to sleep just like we do.

to exploring the potential therapeutic effects of poo, there is evidence from rodent-based studies that faecal transplantation can result in radical changes to both body weight and metabolic status (24). To date, human studies have not yet demonstrated effective weight loss in people with obesity who have received faecal transplants (24, 25). Who knows what the future of poo-based therapy will hold though! Watch this pot.

This chapter has been a story about your poo: if you like, a crap story well told. More specifically, it has been a story about the countless trillions of microbes, the gut microbiota that live and flourish in your poo. We have explored the origins of the gut microbiota and the intricate ways in which the gut microbiota and brain talk to each other. We have discussed the ways in which we can nurture our gut microbiota through lifestyle strategies, to promote our own health and well-being. There is a well-known aphorism that is often used to conclude any literature on the gut microbiota: 'look after them and they will look after you'. I am not going to conclude this chapter with that rather hackneyed statement. Instead, I am going to go one step further and in the process take a lesson from our excessively woke modern-day culture, in which we need to watch our pronouns for fear of causing any offence. In this spirit, we should not refer to our gut microbiota as he, she, them, they or it. Furthermore, our gut microbiota is not some alien being that is parasitising us and eating all our food. Rather, our gut microbiota is part of us and forms an essential organ that is as important for our survival and well-being as our heart or brain. Indeed, our gut microbiota influences our brain activity, emotions and behaviour and, in so doing, makes us who we are. One may even say that our gut microbiota forms an important extension of our brain (which brings a whole new meaning to that well-known insult!). In a similar way to how we need to look after the healthiness of our heart and brain, so too we need to nurture and care for the health and well-being of our gut microbiota. We need to shift our perspective of our gut microbiota from 'they' and 'them' to 'we' and 'us'. Taking ownership of our gut microbiota as a key part of 'us' is a great way to help prevent and manage obesity and promote our own health, well-being and happiness.

References

1. Barber TM, Valsamakis G, Mastorakos G, Hanson P, Kyrou I, Randeva HS, et al. Dietary influences on the microbiota-gut-brain axis. Int J Mol Sci. 2021;22(7):3502.
2. Lozupone CA, Stombaugh JI, Gordon JI, Jansson JK, Knight R. Diversity, stability and resilience of the human gut microbiota. Nature. 2012;489(7415):220–30.
3. Mueller NT, Bakacs E, Combellick J, Grigoryan Z, Dominguez-Bello MG. The infant microbiome development: mom matters. Trends Mol med. 2015;21(2):109–17.
4. Qin J, Li R, Raes J, Arumugam M, Burgdorf KS, Manichanh C, et al. A human gut microbial gene catalogue established by metagenomic sequencing. Nature. 2010;464(7285):59–65.
5. Mayer EA, Tillisch K, Gupta A. Gut/brain axis and the microbiota. J Clin Invest. 2015;125(3):926–38.
6. Barber TM, Kabisch S, Pfeiffer AFH, Weickert MO. The gut microbiome as a key determinant of the heritability of body mass index. Nutrients. 2025;17(10):1713.
7. Bravo JA, Forsythe P, Chew MV, Escaravage E, Savignac HM, Dinan TG, et al. Ingestion of Lactobacillus strain regulates emotional behavior and central GABA receptor expression in a mouse via the vagus nerve. Proc Natl Acad Sci U S A. 2011;108(38):16050–5.
8. Barber TM, Hanson P, Weickert MO. Metabolic-associated fatty liver disease and the gut microbiota. Endocrinol Metab Clin North Am. 2023;52(3):485–96.
9. Neufeld KA, Kang N, Bienenstock J, Foster JA. Effects of intestinal microbiota on anxiety-like behavior. Commun Integr Biol. 2011;4(4):492–4.
10. Bercik P, Denou E, Collins J, Jackson W, Lu J, Jury J, et al. The intestinal microbiota affect central levels of brain-derived neurotropic factor and behavior in mice. Gastroenterology. 2011;141(2):599–609, e1-3.
11. Neufeld KM, Kang N, Bienenstock J, Foster JA. Reduced anxiety-like behavior and central neurochemical change in germ-free mice. Neurogastroenterol Motil. 2011;23(3):255–64, e119.
12. Nishino R, Mikami K, Takahashi H, Tomonaga S, Furuse M, Hiramoto T, et al. Commensal microbiota modulate murine behaviors in a strictly contamination-free environment confirmed by culture-based methods. Neurogastroenterol Motil. 2013;25(6):521–8.

13. Wikoff WR, Anfora AT, Liu J, Schultz PG, Lesley SA, Peters EC, et al. Metabolomics analysis reveals large effects of gut microflora on mammalian blood metabolites. Proc Natl Acad Sci. 2009;106(10):3698–703.
14. Sanmiguel CP, Jacobs J, Gupta A, Ju T, Stains J, Coveleskie K, et al. Surgically induced changes in gut microbiome and hedonic eating as related to weight loss: preliminary findings in obese women undergoing bariatric surgery. Psychosom Med. 2017;79(8):880.
15. Chambers ES, Viardot A, Psichas A, Morrison DJ, Murphy KG, Zac-Varghese SE, et al. Effects of targeted delivery of propionate to the human colon on appetite regulation, body weight maintenance and adiposity in overweight adults. Gut. 2015;64(11):1744–54.
16. Bibbo S, Ianiro G, Giorgio V, Scaldaferri F, Masucci L, Gasbarrini A, et al. The role of diet on gut microbiota composition. Eur Rev Med Pharmacol Sci. 2016;20(22):4742–9.
17. Adler CJ, Dobney K, Weyrich LS, Kaidonis J, Walker AW, Haak W, et al. Sequencing ancient calcified dental plaque shows changes in oral microbiota with dietary shifts of the Neolithic and Industrial revolutions. Nat Genet. 2013;45(4):450–5, 5e1.
18. David LA, Maurice CF, Carmody RN, Gootenberg DB, Button JE, Wolfe BE, et al. Diet rapidly and reproducibly alters the human gut microbiome. Nature. 2014;505(7484):559–63.
19. Barber TM, Kabisch S, Pfeiffer AFH, Weickert MO. The Health Benefits of Dietary Fibre. Nutrients. 2020;12(10).
20. Duca FA, Sakar Y, Covasa M. The modulatory role of high fat feeding on gastrointestinal signals in obesity. J Nutr Biochem. 2013;24(10):1663–77.
21. Hill M. Intestinal flora and endogenous vitamin synthesis. Eur J Cancer Prev. 1997;6:S43–5.
22. Barber TM, Kabisch S, Pfeiffer AFH, Weickert MO. Dietary and lifestyle strategies for obesity. Nutrients. 2024;16(16):2714.
23. Kim KO, Gluck M. Fecal microbiota transplantation: an update on clinical practice. Clin Endosc. 2019;52(2):137.
24. Lee P, Yacyshyn BR, Yacyshyn MB. Gut microbiota and obesity: an opportunity to alter obesity through faecal microbiota transplant (FMT). Diabetes Obes Metab. 2019;21(3):479–90.
25. Kootte RS, Levin E, Salojarvi J, Smits LP, Hartstra AV, Udayappan SD, et al. Improvement of insulin sensitivity after lean donor feces in metabolic syndrome is driven by baseline intestinal microbiota composition. Cell Metab. 2017;26(4):611–9 e6.

6 Sleep as a Pillar of Health

There is an Irish proverb that says 'a good laugh and a long sleep are the best cures in the doctor's book' (1). Having worked as a doctor in the NHS for the last 27 years and managed tens of thousands of patients, I tend to agree with this. The best therapies are often non-pharmacological. Social interaction, sharing a joke and getting good amounts of restful sleep are indeed therapeutic and often cathartic. We should not underestimate their healing powers. For many of us, sleep is an activity that we spend more time doing than any other. We may spend perhaps between 20–33% of our lives asleep. There is a good reason for this. We need our sleep! During sleep, our brains are literally cleansed of all the gunk (there is a medical term for it, but let's not get bogged down with medical jargon) that is deposited within our neurons during waking hours: a kind of internal washing machine for the brain, switched on during sleep. Furthermore, pretty much every aspect of our physiology requires restful sleep of sufficient duration to function normally. Disturbances to our sleep duration, quality or pattern can contribute to chronic illness, including Cardiovascular disease (CVD), mental health problems and even dementia, to name but a few. Sleep is important for memory formation and essential for our emotional regulation, our psychosocial interactions and our executive function: how well we can plan our lives and deal with the daily stresses and strains of living that we all face. It turns out that sleep is also important for our metabolic health and body weight, the focus of this chapter. I will discuss initially the negative impact of our modern-day obesogenic environment on our sleep and the mechanisms that link our sleep with the control of our appetite and metabolism. (I use the term 'obesogenic' to refer to an environment that promotes weight gain and the development of obesity, discussed further in the last chapter.) I will then outline strategies for us to optimise our sleep duration, quality and pattern as an essential component of a healthy lifestyle.

The Negative Impact of Our Modern-Day Obesogenic Environment on Our Sleep

How much sleep do you get each night (or each day if you work night shifts)? How restful is your sleep? Is your sleep disturbed? Is your sleep-wake cycle constant each night and day? These are important questions that we should all ask ourselves. Unfortunately, it seems that our modern-day world has caused disruption to our sleep. Many of us are sleep deprived. Average sleep duration has diminished over the last century (2). In the early 20th century, average sleep duration each night for adults living in the Western world was around 9 hours. Imagine that! It would be like going to sleep at 10 pm and then waking at 7 am the next day. How many of us get this amount of sleep each night? Not many, I suspect. By the 1980s, average nightly sleep duration dropped to 7 hours (1, 3). Since the 1980s, there has been a further decline in our sleep duration, with 30% of adults having <7 hours each night in 2010 (1, 3). It is estimated that between 9–24% of the population suffers from excessive daytime sleepiness due to sleep deprivation (1). However, even if you don't feel sleepy during the day, you may still be sleep deprived. Sleep experts recommend that as adults, we should all be getting around 7.5 hours of sleep per night. My wrist-worn 'health-tracker' tells me that my mean average sleeping duration this year is 7 hours, 18 minutes, and so even I am sleep deprived by an average of 12 minutes per night, based on expert recommendation.

There are multiple factors that may scupper our sleep duration, quality and pattern. Our modern-day world seems to place increased demands on our time. We live in a '24-hour society', in which we have instant access to services and provisions, all available to us through our personal electronic devices (1). Rather than going to a travel agent during waking hours, we can now book our next holiday or train ticket online at 3 am. Much of our interactions with the world and with others now play out in an online virtual world and can be conducted at any time, including during the night. Accordingly, our daily lives are less well punctuated than they were decades ago. Growing up as a child, I remember at around 12 am when the BBC had completed that day's television transmissions, there would be a patriotic rendition of the national anthem followed by an irritating loud and high-pitched monotone accompanied by a little white dot in the middle of the screen. At this point in the daily proceedings, the only thing to do was to switch the TV off and go to bed. There was literally nothing else to do (apart from reading a book, perhaps). The world had closed itself down for the day, and sleep was now on the agenda (*fig 6.1*). This was satirised hilariously in the 1980s sitcom '*The*

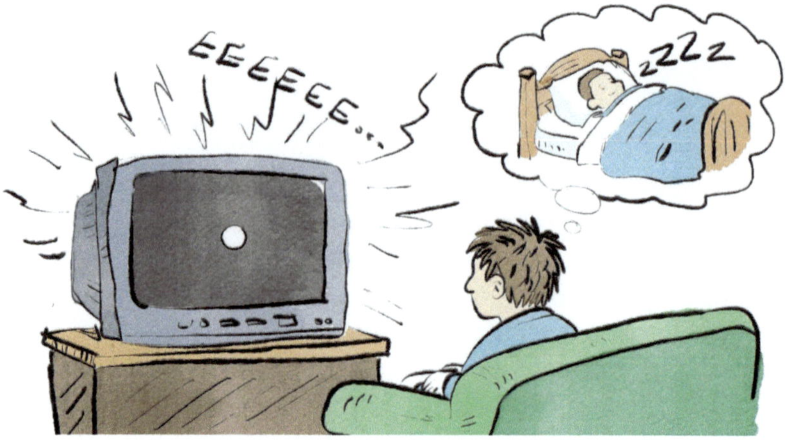

Figure 6.1: Punctuated day/night transition in our pre-information revolution world.

Young Ones', in which Rick asked what the little white dot means, to which Neil replied that 'it means something really heavy, it means that it is time to go to bed'. When Vivyan continued to watch the little white dot, a guard suddenly appeared on screen, telling him to 'go to bed, spotty!' Ah, those were the days. The golden age of television, before video, internet, multi-channel 24/7 TV and streaming services. How times have changed! Now, there is no equivalent of the little white dot in the middle of the screen and the high-pitched monotone, punctuating clearly a transition between day and night. If sleep was not an essential biological function, we could easily spend our lives in 'waking-mode' 24 hours a day in today's world. But not back then.

In addition to our modern-day lack of day/night external punctuation, our availability as individuals has transformed radically in recent times (2). Our personal electronic devices follow us everywhere we go, and they seem to have become an extension of us, like an additional appendage. Many of us may feel lost without them, almost like losing an arm or a leg. These devices are now ubiquitous and may even follow us to bed. With all its benefits and advantages, our modern-day highly connected and '24-hour instant access' society has created an unprecedented intrusiveness into our daily lives. Rather than being cherished 'me time' that is free from interruption and intrusion, our modern-day environment creates the potential to distract us during the night and thereby to disrupt our sleep (2). Finally, a lack of clear external punctuation of our 24-hour cycles of night and day also means that we are less likely to achieve a regular sleep-wake cycle, with consistent sleeping and waking times each night and day, as recommended by sleep experts.

Mechanisms That Link Our Sleep with the Control of Appetite and Metabolism

As intimated earlier, sleep deprivation negatively affects virtually every aspect of our physiology and is linked to the development of chronic illness and even premature mortality (1). In Chapter 2, I discussed the control of our appetite and the many factors that can influence that control. I also described our appetite control as having a 'seesaw' relationship with the control of metabolism, mediated by the melanocortin 4 (MC4) receptor: when one is up, the other is down and vice versa. I described two dimmer switches that regulate our appetite, one up-switch and one down-switch. It turns out that regular restful sleep of a sufficient duration is important for the proper regulation of our appetite and metabolism and therefore our body weight and overall predisposition to obesity. To use the dimmer switch analogy, our sleep provides the oil and lubrication for these switches to function normally, and when we are sleep deprived, our appetite dimmer switches don't work as well, with the result of enhanced appetite and diminished metabolic rate (how many kcals we burn each night and day through our metabolism).

There is a clear and well-established link between our sleep and the control of appetite and metabolism, with data derived from diverse origins, including epidemiological, animal- and human-based studies (4). In a nutshell, when we are sleep deprived, there are changes to the levels of hormones in our blood that regulate our appetite and metabolism. These include hormones like ghrelin that enhance our appetite (and suppress metabolism) and leptin and insulin that both help to suppress appetite (and enhance metabolism), contingent upon the sensitivities of their respective receptors (4). These hormones are released from the periphery and act centrally on the appetite up- and down-dimmer switches within the hypothalamus to mediate these changes in appetite and metabolism. In one human-based study, the levels of ghrelin and leptin in the blood were explored in healthy young men and compared between the contexts of sleep sufficiency and sleep deprivation. In this study, just 2 nights of sleep restriction resulted in a significant reduction in the blood levels of leptin and a significant increase in the blood levels of ghrelin (5). As a result of these changes in the hormones that regulate the appetite dimmer switches, sleep restriction resulted in an enhancement of hunger and appetite and an increased intake of calories, especially calorie-dense foods with a high content of carbohydrate (5). In addition to adverse effects on the control of our appetite and metabolism, sleep deprivation can also contribute towards the development of insulin resistance (6), a forerunner of metabolic dysfunction, including Type 2 Diabetes Mellitus.

Strategies to Optimise Our Sleep Duration, Quality and Pattern

Why all the fuss about sleep? Can't we just ignore our sleep and focus on diet and exercise? What does it matter that we get less sleep than our parents and grandparents had? Traditionally, public health messages regarding healthy lifestyles (and by implication our propensity for weight gain and the development of obesity) have focused predominantly on the two main pillars of lifestyle, diet and exercise. Indeed, many of my patients who live with obesity seem surprised when I ask them about their sleep, when they see me for their initial clinical assessments. Sleep seems to have been hidden from view, a forgotten relative. Indeed, sleep is a somewhat forgotten area of healthcare and has been neglected for decades. It is perhaps more convenient for us to ignore our sleep and to focus on what seem like the important things, the events that occupy our waking lives. This is unfortunate given the essential role that sleep plays for our health and for our ability to deal with the events that occupy our waking lives. It is my belief that sleep justifiably deserves its own pillar alongside diet and exercise. Rather than being hidden away, this pillar of sleep should assume a position of prominence, a pillar that trumps all else and one that demands the regular focus and attention of all of us (*fig 6.2*). If we can use the analogy of a house to represent our waking lives (including all that we do, say, think, feel, believe, plan, interact and know), we can liken our sleep to the very foundations of that house. Hidden away from view but nonetheless forming an essential role, foundation and scaffold on which our daily wakeful lives depend. Furthermore, although not proven, it seems likely that the sleep deprivation

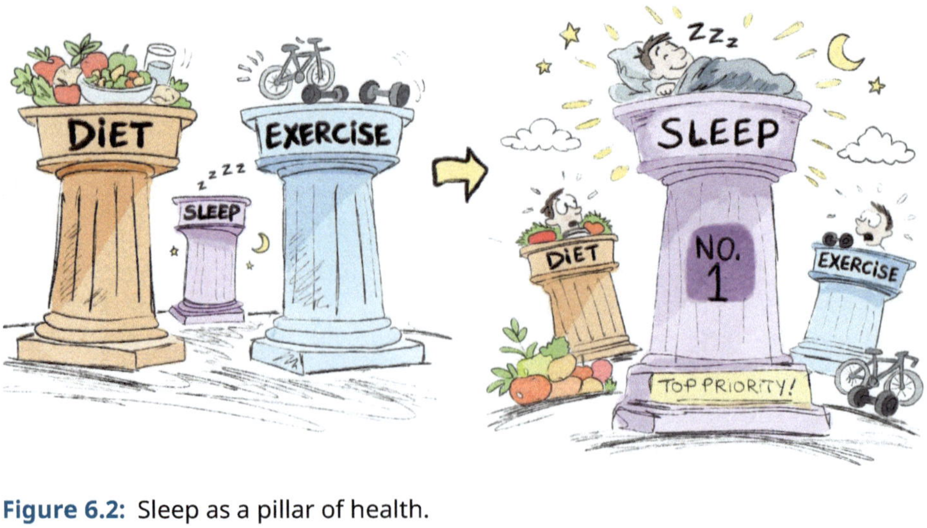

Figure 6.2: Sleep as a pillar of health.

that typifies our modern-day society is a likely contributor to the global obesity problem.

Unsurprisingly, sleep deprivation stymies our ability to adopt healthy lifestyles during our waking lives, including dietary modification. In one study on overweight adults, the effects of 2 weeks of moderate caloric restriction on body composition were compared between a scenario of sleep sufficiency (8.5 hours of sleep per night) and that of sleep deprivation (5.5 hours of sleep per night) in the same participants. Compared with sleep sufficiency, sleep deprivation reduced the ability to lose fat mass (by 55%) and increased the loss of lean body mass such as skeletal muscle (by 60%) (7). Therefore, body composition was impaired during caloric restriction when sleep deprived. Sleep restriction also resulted in enhanced hunger and reduced fat oxidation (7). It follows that the success of any weight loss attempts through dietary change (or indeed the adoption of healthy diet generally to prevent weight gain and obesity) depends upon the sufficiency of our sleep. Put simply, our ability to adopt healthy lifestyles, and the health benefits of such strategies, are both contingent upon the duration and quality of our sleep. For any healthy lifestyle approach, addressing our sleep should be the first step. Our sleep forms an essential component of any discussion on obesity, its pathogenesis and its effective prevention and management.

In recent times, we have witnessed a renaissance in our understanding of and focus on sleep in healthcare (8). Based on recent evidence and insights, we have a greater understanding now regarding the importance of our sleep for our health and well-being, and the status of sleep as an important pillar of healthy lifestyle is slowly emerging from the mist.

As alluded to earlier, there are three aspects of our sleep that we should each address. The first is sleep duration. This is not the amount of time that we spend in bed, but rather the amount of time that we spend asleep. The National Institutes of Health recommends that as adults, we should sleep for between 7 and 8 hours each night (1, 9). I appreciate that this is a tall order for many of us. There may be valid reasons that prevent some of us from achieving this recommendation, possibly the care of babies and young children or the care of relatives who need our attention during the night. Maybe our jobs interfere with the amount of sleep that we can get, maybe we suffer from chronic pain that keeps us awake at night, or maybe we just find it difficult to sleep for that duration. Some of us suffer from insomnia, and this of course can severely limit sleep duration. However, in many of us, achieving between 7 and 8 hours of sleep each night may be entirely possible. Each of us needs to explore the many factors in our own lives that may prevent us from getting sufficient sleep duration each night (some of these factors I have discussed in this chapter) and then consider how these could be addressed in a way that enables longer sleep duration. We may not achieve the recommended >7 hours sleep each night, but even if we can improve our sleep duration from, say, 5 to 6 hours per night, this would have important favorable effects on our health generally. This would also facilitate the proper regulation of our appetite and metabolism and therefore help us to maintain a healthy body weight and composition.

The second important aspect of our sleep is its quality. This is more difficult to quantify than sleep duration. A 'health-tracker' may struggle to do this, although some may provide a sleep quality score. Our sleep quality may vary each night. We can all relate to how worries, anxieties and stress can impact on the restfulness of our sleep. Getting off to sleep becomes more difficult when we are anxious about something, and we may be more prone to wake up from our sleep or have nightmares if we are stressed and anxious. This is all part of being human! (Incidentally, I learnt recently that the term 'nightmare' has nothing to do with horses, but rather comes from the Old English word 'mare' that refers to a mythological demon or goblin that sits on the chest and torments us whilst we sleep.) The experience of pain or the need to get up and pass urine frequently during the night (nocturia) can also impair the quality of our sleep. If you experience these symptoms, you should speak to your doctor (in men, the latter can indicate a problem with your prostate, and in all of us, nocturia can be a sign of Diabetes Mellitus). Furthermore, some of us may suffer from conditions like 'Obstructive Sleep Apnoea' (OSA) which itself is related to obesity, and results in recurrent apnoeic episodes during the night. ('Apnoea' is when our breathing stops for at least 10 seconds.) OSA increases the risk of CVD and other chronic illnesses. OSA often improves with effective weight loss and can present with increased sleepiness during the day, morning headaches and troublesome hypertension (elevated blood pressure). OSA is under-diagnosed. If you are concerned that you may have OSA or if your sleeping partner reports that you stop breathing recurrently during the night, you should see your doctor and get it checked out. If necessary, you should be referred to a sleep centre for appropriate investigation, diagnosis and management of sleep-related disorders such as OSA and/or insomnia (that often coexists with OSA) that may impact negatively on your sleep duration and/or quality and your metabolic health (10). Beyond the diagnosis and effective management of conditions like OSA and insomnia, there are strategies that we can all adopt to improve the quality of our sleep, some of which may seem obvious. The main principles of good sleep hygiene are outlined here:

Dark: Darkness enables us to release melatonin naturally, a hormone that facilitates sleep and promotes 'quiet wakefulness'. If there is too much ambient light in our bedroom, then this is sensed by the retina, and this can impair the release of melatonin and confuse the brain regarding the timing of the sleep-wake cycle. Put simply, our brain is programmed to sleep when it is dark, not when it is light. You may think that closing your eyes solves this problem, but you would be wrong. There are light-sensitive cells within the retina that signal to the brain the presence of ambient light, even when our eyes are closed. So, make sure your bedroom is dark. Furthermore, during the hour or two before you go to sleep, ensure that you are in a relatively dark environment to enable you to produce melatonin naturally. Avoid 'blue light' exposure from screens before bedtime, and if you have a dimmer switch on your lights, you could turn them down. Reading a book with a dimmed light can help.

Quiet: It is difficult to sleep in a noisy environment. For restful sleep, the brain needs peace and quiet. For those of us who live in a big city with 24/7 ambient noise, achieving a peaceful nocturnal environment may be easier said than done. If we experience noise at night, we should explore ways in which this could be mitigated against. Simple measures like closing the bedroom door or having a quiet 'word' with night-time noise creators who may share your house, flat or other accommodation may work. Thicker curtains to block out ambient noise from the outside could be another measure. There may be aspects of our noise environment though that we simply cannot change. You can't very easily stop the traffic from trundling past your house at night!

Cool: When we sleep, our body temperature drops by around 1°C. This is one reason why it is harder to sleep in a hot environment. At the time of writing, the United Kingdom had just experienced its hottest summer on record, with four separate heatwaves during the summer of 2025. Tropical nights, when the minimum temperature does not fall below 20°C, can make sleeping difficult. At other times of the year, we can adjust the temperature control in our bedrooms, making them slightly cooler than the rest of the house, to facilitate sleep. During hot summers, simple measures like opening the window at night, use of a fan, and shutting blinds and curtains during the day can help. Immersing our hands in cold water and splashing cool water on the face and head can also help to cool down body temperature before going to sleep (*fig 6.3*).

Conditioning: By this, I am not referring to what you put on your hair following shampooing. (Being bald, this is an alien concept to me.) Rather, I mean it is important to condition the brain, so it learns what the bed is for. Conducting one's day-time activities during waking hours from one's bed is generally a bad idea (excepting, of course, the infamous 'Bed-In for Peace' staged by John Lennon and Yoko Ono in 1969). To do so confuses the brain regarding the purpose of the bed.

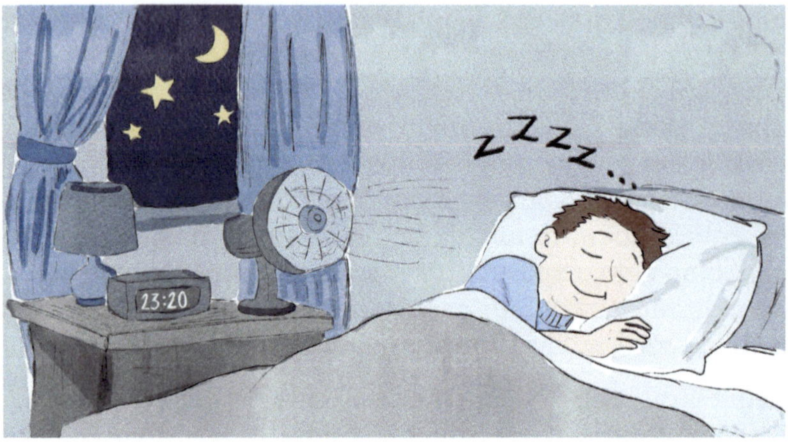

Figure 6.3: The ideal sleeping environment.

Reserve the bed for sleeping. And perhaps one other activity that we won't mention here. Otherwise, conduct your day-time activities during waking hours out of bed and ideally outside of the bedroom.

Routine: It is hard to overstate the importance of routine for restful sleep. In the same way that the brain is conditioned to sleep in bed, so too it is conditioned for a regular sleep-wake cycle. Although natural biological processes occur that help to establish a 'diurnal' (daily 24-hour) cycle, there are things that we can all do to help entrain and optimise this process. Exposure to natural light on waking in the morning helps to regulate our normal sleep-wake cycle, in a similar way to the avoidance of bright light exposure in the hours before sleep. Try to avoid meals in the couple of hours before sleep, as the process of active digestion and assimilation of nutrients can make sleep more difficult. Similarly, the avoidance of strenuous exercise in the couple of hours before sleep is important. However, engagement in physical activity and exercise during the day is facilitative of restful sleep. This may seem paradoxical, but being sedentary all day impairs our ability to enjoy restful sleep. Conversely, being physically tired from engaging in exercise during the day improves our sleep. Try to eat regular meals and eat healthily: our nutrition influences our overall well-being that in turn impacts on our sleep duration and quality (11). In short, our diet influences our sleep and vice versa. If we have regular restful sleep of sufficient duration, this empowers us to deal more effectively with the inevitable stresses and strains of daily living. In a virtuous circle, this in turn will facilitate further restful sleep.

There are a few other important points regarding routine. Try to avoid ingestion of caffeine beyond early afternoon. Try to restrict this to the morning if you can, as caffeine can have a delayed response that can impair sleep if drunk later in the day. Although alcohol is a sedative and therefore may be assumed to improve one's sleep, it impairs the quality of sleep, so avoid excessive alcohol generally, and particularly before sleep. Try to avoid sleeping pills as these worsen sleep quality. If you are struggling to get to sleep, avoid looking at your watch or clock, as this can result in time anxiety. Instead, get up and read something in dim light until you feel sleepy. This will have an added benefit of taking your mind off whatever it was that was causing anxiety and preventing you from falling asleep. And finally, if your electronic device must follow you to bed, think of ways in which its intrusiveness can be limited, through silencing its pings for example, to facilitate more restful sleep.

The final important aspect of our sleep is related to routine: pattern. This means the timing of our sleep. We could get 7.5 hours of restful sleep in every 24-hour cycle, but if the timing of this sleep is widely variable, and sometimes occurs during the day, and at other times during the night, this is not necessarily favorable for our health. For some of us who work shifts or who may be unable to get regular and sufficient sleep during the night for other reasons, I empathise. A regular sleeping pattern may simply not be possible. However, for many of us, it should be possible to strive for a regular sleeping pattern. Sleep experts advise that our sleeping and waking times should be around the same times every night and day, including at weekends. For those of us who like a lie-in at the weekends (including myself on occasions), I appreciate this is not what you might want to hear. But just as with bed-conditioning and punctuation of our lives with a regular routine, the brain also responds well to a regular sleep-wake cycle. One caveat to mention here is that our natural sleep-wake cycle may change as we age. Notoriously, teenagers often have a predilection for late bedtimes and late wake-up times, and in older people we often see the reverse of this. Furthermore, each of us has individual preferences (as 'owls' or 'larks') regarding the timing of our bedtimes and waking times. However, the important point to make across all these scenarios is that whatever our usual and preferred bedtime and waking times are, we try to stick to the same sleeping and waking routine and times every night and day (*fig 6.4*).

There are many aspects of our physiology, including our endocrine (hormonal) regulation that play out on a 24-hour diurnal sleep-wake cycle, and if this is disrupted, then this can have adverse effects on our metabolic and overall health. In the last chapter, we learnt about the importance of our gut microbiota for our health. We also learnt about the importance of allowing our gut microbiota sufficient time to sleep. Incredibly, it turns out that our gut microbiota has its own sleep-wake

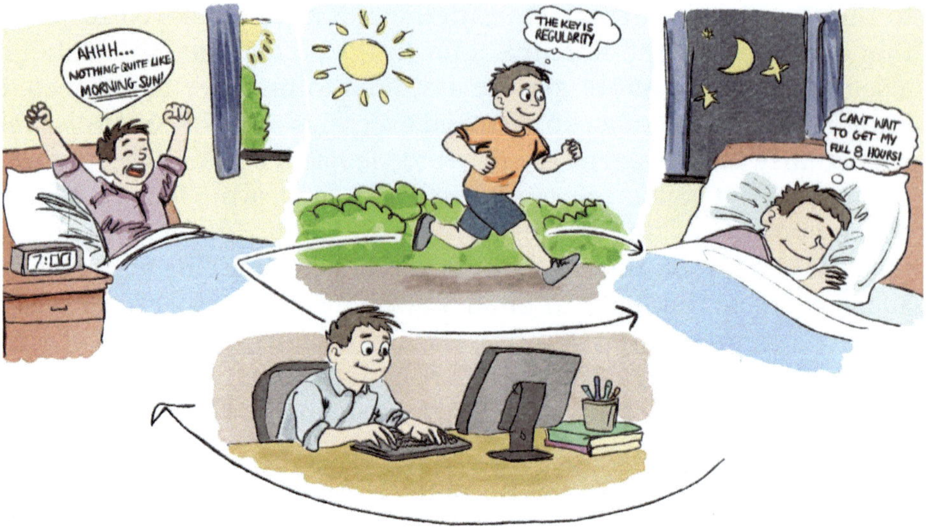

Figure 6.4: A regular sleep-wake cycle.

cycle (12): our gut microbiota sleeps when we do! The sleep-wake cycle of our gut microbiota helps to entrain our own sleep-wake cycle and vice versa. And just like us, our gut microbiota also dislikes being disturbed during sleeping time and to do so negatively impacts on our metabolic health. Let sleeping gut microbiota lie!

There is one other final point to make regarding the importance of a regular sleep-wake cycle and routine. During our waking hours, there is a clock within our brain which ticks away. The longer we are awake, the more tired and fatigued we feel: the so-called 'sleep pressure' (the body's natural urge to sleep). After 12-hours of being awake, we start to feel significantly more tired and fatigued. It follows that if we lie in for a few hours on a Saturday morning, we won't feel as tired at our usual bedtime on a Saturday evening and may find it more difficult to get to sleep. This can then have an adverse knock-on effect for the next day (and potentially the following week), especially in the context of alcohol intake on a Saturday evening, which can also impair our sleep quality. When all is said and done, it is best to stick to the same sleeping and waking times every night and day, for both working and leisure days.

So much for the well-recited (and slightly irritating) mantra for obesity management that is 'eat less, move more'. Surely 'sleep more, sleep well and sleep regularly' is a more meaningful mantra that we can all aspire to. And with that, as it is 22.13 at the time of writing, I think it is time for some sufficient, restful and correctly timed sleep, but not before I switch off my laptop, dim the lights, read a book....

References

1. Liew SC, Aung T. Sleep deprivation and its association with diseases – a review. Sleep Med. 2021;77:192–204.
2. Barber TM, Kabisch S, Pfeiffer AFH, Weickert MO. Dietary and lifestyle strategies for obesity. Nutrients. 2024;16(16):2714.
3. Schoenborn CA, Adams PE. Health behaviors of adults: United States, 2005-2007. Vital Health Stat 10. 2010;(245):1–132.
4. Liu S, Wang X, Zheng Q, Gao L, Sun Q. Sleep deprivation and central appetite regulation. Nutrients. 2022;14(24):5196.
5. Spiegel K, Tasali E, Penev P, Van Cauter E. Brief communication: sleep curtailment in healthy young men is associated with decreased leptin levels, elevated ghrelin levels, and increased hunger and appetite. Ann Intern Med. 2004;141(11):846–50.
6. Singh P, Beyl RA, Stephens JM, Noland RC, Richard AJ, Boudreau A, et al. Effect of sleep restriction on insulin sensitivity and energy metabolism in postmenopausal women: a randomized crossover trial. Obesity (Silver Spring). 2023;31(5):1204–15.
7. Nedeltcheva AV, Kilkus JM, Imperial J, Schoeller DA, Penev PD. Insufficient sleep undermines dietary efforts to reduce adiposity. Ann Intern Med. 2010;153(7):435–41.
8. Soong C, Burry L, Cho HJ, Gathecha E, Kisuule F, Tannenbaum C, et al. An implementation guide to promote sleep and reduce sedative-hypnotic initiation for noncritically Ill inpatients. JAMA Intern Med. 2019;179(7):965–72.
9. Luyster FS, Strollo PJ Jr, Zee PC, Walsh JK. Boards of Directors of the American Academy of Sleep M, the Sleep Research S. Sleep: a health imperative. Sleep. 2012;35(6):727–34.
10. Duan D, Kim LJ, Jun JC, Polotsky VY. Connecting insufficient sleep and insomnia with metabolic dysfunction. Ann N Y Acad Sci. 2023;1519(1):94–117.
11. Zhao M, Tuo H, Wang S, Zhao L. The effects of dietary nutrition on sleep and sleep disorders. Mediators Inflamm. 2020;2020:3142874.
12. Pang X, Chen L, Xu G. New awareness of the interplay between the gut microbiota and circadian rhythms. Pol J Microbiol. 2023;72(4):355–63.

7 Physical Exercise

Ah yes, physical exercise! Love it or loathe it, we can't ignore it, and any book on obesity would be remiss without its inclusion. Physical exercise and diet are like a couple who have been happily married for over 50-years, inextricably linked and firmly bonded as two sentinel-like pillars of healthy lifestyle. As with diet, there are many misconceptions when it comes to its wedded partner physical exercise. Furthermore, the term 'physical exercise' has become so hackneyed, and we are so used to hearing it that we may gloss over in our minds its true meaning and utility.

In its simplest form, physical exercise refers to us using our skeletal muscles (SMs). Broadly, physical exercise comes in two main forms. The first, so-called 'cardiovascular' exercise, involves use of SMs in a way that requires enhanced cardiovascular work, with increased heart and breathing rates, for example. By using our SMs in this way, metabolic rate increases (due to the increased work of the SMs), and this in turn requires increased cardiovascular work (that further increases metabolic rate) to support this increased metabolism. Physical exercises like running, rowing and walking are examples of such 'cardiovascular' exercise. The second form of physical exercise, 'resistance' exercise (or 'training'), involves contracting SMs against resistance. Lifting weights would be one example. Resistance training still requires increased cardiovascular work, but not usually as much as for cardiovascular exercise. Ideally, when we engage in physical exercise, we should incorporate both these exercise types into our regime. Generally, cardiovascular exercise helps to improve our physical fitness that in turn has a major beneficial impact on our overall metabolic health, mortality and expected lifespan. Conversely, resistance training helps to build and maintain our SM mass that in turn optimises our metabolic efficiency, as discussed in Chapter 4.

Another way of stratifying physical exercise is through its intensity. In this regard, there is quite a large spectrum that extends all the way from 'couch potato-esque' sedentariness at one extreme to 'high-intensity interval training' (HIIT) at the other extreme and everything in between. One problem of using the term 'physical exercise' is that it usually evokes

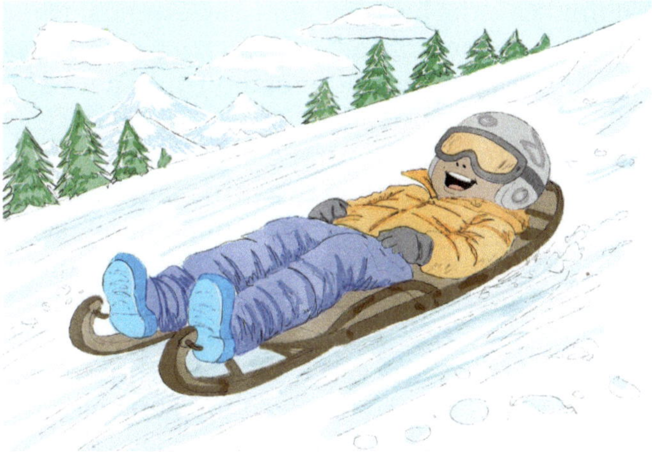

Figure 7.1: The luge.

visions of someone working and sweating it out on a treadmill or cross trainer. As outlined, this form of physical exercise is quite specific. A better term would be 'physical activity' as this umbrella term incorporates any form of SM work, cardiovascular or resistance and regardless of intensity. Essentially, any activity that is non-sedentary. Accordingly, I will use the term 'physical activity' for the rest of this chapter. At this point, we should also define sedentariness as any activity that involves sitting or lying during waking hours. This is except perhaps the 'luge', a winter Olympics sport that admittedly does involve lying down on one's back, but I would imagine is also quite physically strenuous (*fig 7.1*).

With that preamble, in this chapter, I will focus on three main aspects of physical activity (physical activity and metabolic rate, the truth about sedentariness and the metabolic benefits of physical activity), whilst addressing some common misconceptions. To conclude the chapter, I will provide some suggestions regarding the optimisation of physical activity in any healthy lifestyle program.

Physical Activity and Metabolic Rate

Whenever I am interviewed by the national media on obesity-related topics, one question that is guaranteed to come up is 'What's the best way to speed up our metabolism?' Within our collective psyche, we seem to have internalised a model in which our metabolic rates can be sped up or slowed down at will and that this simple act of adjusting our metabolic rate then translates into meaningful changes in our body weight. If only that were true, and if it were as simple as that! The reality is that, as with any other aspect of our biology, our metabolic rate is a fundamental aspect of our physiology and has complex regulatory pathways that implicate the hypothalamus, an essential part of the brain that helps to keep us on the strait and narrow in so many ways, including the regulation of our appetite and metabolism. There are drug therapies in development that can speed up our metabolism. In fact, the first ever weight loss drug (2,4-Dinitrophenol, DNP) that was popular in the early 20th century was based on this principle. However, just as the other use of DNP in explosives can result in fatalities, so too did DNP used for weight loss (through hyperthermia, a condition in which the body overheats from an over-revved metabolism, akin to your car engine overheating and giving up the ghost when there is no coolant on a hot day), and this led to its withdrawal. We should learn from this. Rather than asking 'what's the best way to speed up metabolism?', we should understand that our metabolism is not something to be messed with or tinkered with. Having said this, drug therapies that can help to speed up metabolism in a very controlled way do have potential therapeutic utility, and this is explored further in Chapter 10.

When it comes to physical activity, a common belief is that this is an excellent way to speed up metabolism, to burn off calories in the process and thereby to help with weight loss. That physical activity increases our metabolic rate is indubitably true. It is logical that if we work our SMs harder, this will increase demand for a fuel supply (primarily glucose and lipids) and oxygen via the blood for these working muscles, and metabolic rate will increase. It is also true that this process will likely help with any lifestyle program that facilitates weight loss or the prevention of weight gain (including weight maintenance). This much is true. However, we overestimate the strength of this relationship between physical activity and metabolism. It is important to understand that our metabolism is mainly influenced by so-called 'basal metabolic rate' (BMR), which is the energy required to power all our cells. BMR happens all the time, even when we are asleep. As I discussed in Chapter 4, our SM mass is an important determinant of our BMR, even when we are sedentary, as SM is metabolically active even when at rest. When we start to engage in physical activity, our metabolic rate goes up, but not substantially. Furthermore, when it comes to physical activity and metabolism, we tend to suffer from an affliction that affects the human mind, that of 'linearity'. In short, this refers to the idea that the more physical activity we do, the more calories we burn and the greater our metabolic rate, that the duration and intensity of our physical activity correlates directly with metabolic rate and that one is commensurate with the other (1): If I run 10 km on the treadmill, then I will burn twice as many calories as if I run 5 km on the treadmill. We may not even stop to consider whether this way of thinking is accurate. It turns out that it is not.

What happens in reality is that a 'constrained' model links physical activity with our metabolism (1). Evidence for such insights comes from a fascinating study that compared daily metabolic rates between people with Westernised, relatively sedentary lifestyles (people like me and probably like you) and those from African hunter-gatherer tribes (who may think nothing of walking 10 miles each day). This revealed that daily metabolic rates in our species are more constant and less dependent on differences in daily physical activity than previously believed (2, 3). Other studies that have looked at the metabolic rates of people training for a marathon confirm the notion of a constrained model of metabolism, in which increasing levels of physical activity have diminishing incremental effects on metabolic rate, until eventually a plateau is reached, at which any additional physical activity has no further meaningful effect on further increasing metabolic rate (2, 3). When you think about it, it is a good thing that our metabolism adopts a constrained response to physical activity, otherwise if we did nothing but exercise all day, our metabolic rate would go through the roof and may lead to our demise (*fig 7.2*). For this model to work and for a plateaued metabolic rate to be reached with physical activity, there must be some other aspect of metabolism that is 'dumbed down' in response to excessive physical exercise. What this is, how the metabolic plateau is controlled and how this varies according to age, sex and other physiological states and over time in the same person, remain incompletely understood and important research questions (1).

To summarise this section, our overall metabolic rate (number of calories burnt each day) is influenced much less by physical activity than what people think. As a species, our daily metabolic rates are quite similar regardless of whether we are hunter-gatherers who walk 10 miles every day to hunt and collect food, or whether we are Western 'couch potatoes' who rely on the click of a button and a delivery driver to source our food. Of course, physical activity does increase our metabolic rate

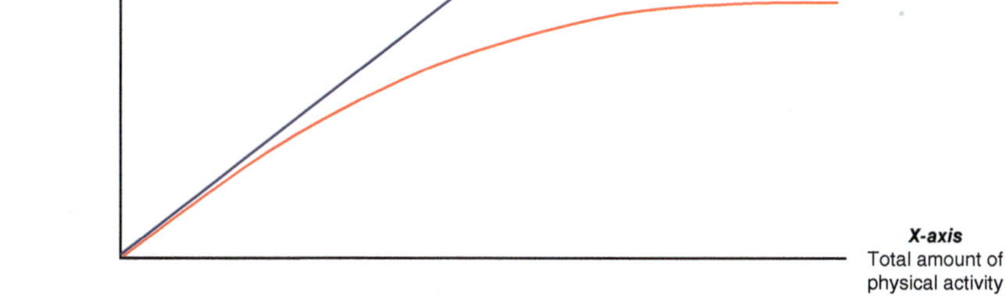

Figure 7.2: Linear versus constrained models of metabolism. The lines show two relationships between total amount of physical activity in any given time (a product of intensity and duration). The blue and red lines show schematic representations of linear and constrained models of metabolism, respectively.

to some degree, but there is a law of diminishing returns when it comes to the relationship between physical activity and metabolic rate. Once a plateau is reached, no amount of additional physical activity will further increase metabolic rate and burn additional calories.

The Truth About Sedentariness

Compared with African hunter-gatherer tribes and perhaps with the exception of elite athletes, we are sedentary. How many hours each day are you sedentary? If you include sleeping time, the answer will probably be most of the time. As with physical activity, sedentariness within our population adopts a spectrum that is inversely related to physical activity: the more physically active you are, the less sedentary and vice versa. Many jobs (including mine) are executed in a sitting (sedentary) position. If you have a job that involves standing (or walking), then at least you are not sedentary at work! Leisure activities like watching television or a film are usually conducted in the sitting position. Sedentariness is often blamed as one of the contributors to the global obesity problem. It is certainly true that modern-day technologies have reduced our need to do physical work, and our lives are now more comfortable and less physically effortful than they were a century ago. However, I would argue that the rise of gym culture and other initiatives such as 'parkrun' and the like have helped to improve our physical activity at least during our leisure time and mitigate against our propensity for technology-induced sedentariness in our modern-day world.

Prolonged sedentariness is bad for our health. Sitting or lying for long periods (except for sleep) increases our risk of premature death. In recent times, the cardiovascular risk of sedentariness (sitting) has even been equated with smoking. This is likely an overexaggeration, with one meta-analysis showing that sedentariness increases the relative risk of dying by around 22%, compared with smoking that nearly triples the risk of dying (with heavy smoking having an even greater effect on mortality) (4). At this point, you may reasonably think that if sedentariness adopts the inverse proportion of physical activity that one reason for the cardiovascular risk of sedentariness stems from its association with lack of physical activity. I agree! However, evidence also suggests that sedentariness per se has an independent effect on cardiovascular risk. Importantly, it is not so much the total duration of sedentariness that matters for our health, but rather whether and how we punctuate prolonged sedentariness. This is good news for those of us who have jobs that involve prolonged sitting!

The regular punctuation of prolonged sedentariness with light physical activities can transform our overall metabolic health. In one study on men with overweight and obesity, uninterrupted sitting for 8.5-hours was compared amongst the same participants with the same duration of sitting but with interruptions every 45-minutes for either a 3-minute walk or 10 squats. This simple measure of regular punctuation of prolonged sitting with light physical activity every 45-minutes resulted in significant improvements in metabolic status, including improved blood sugar control (5). If you work in an open plan office, and you see your work colleague getting up every 45-minutes to do a few squats in the corner, then go and join them! If no one else is doing it, then why not start a new trend? It seems like a small price to pay to improve your cardiovascular health and overall life expectancy, and the increased blood flow will probably make you feel better too, and improve concentration. The avoidance of sedentariness has even been shown to have a beneficial effect on cognitive decline with age and therefore risk for developing dementia (6).

Avoiding sedentariness (or at least punctuating it regularly with a few minutes of light physical activity) may not have a huge impact on your body weight. However, it will have transformative effects on your cardiometabolic health, reduce your risk of dementia and improve your life expectancy. Our modern-day Western culture with its emphasis on computerisation is far removed from the hunter-gatherer lifestyles of our hominid ancestors and cousins who still practice this lifestyle even to this day. Since the Industrial Revolution, we have gradually regressed and transitioned from bipedalism to 'bibuttockism'. Environmental change, which I discuss in Chapter 12, can only go so far to encourage us to be more physically active. Realistically, we are not going to go back to hunter-gatherer status, at least not any time soon. We need to accept that sedentariness is an integral part of our modern-day Westernised environments and lifestyles. However, we can all strive to be more physically active and to punctuate prolonged sedentariness with light physical activities. The key message is that we do not need to climb Mount Everest to achieve this goal. Very simple measures that we can all adopt into our daily lives and would not even break us out into a sweat can and do work metabolic wonders (*fig 7.3*).

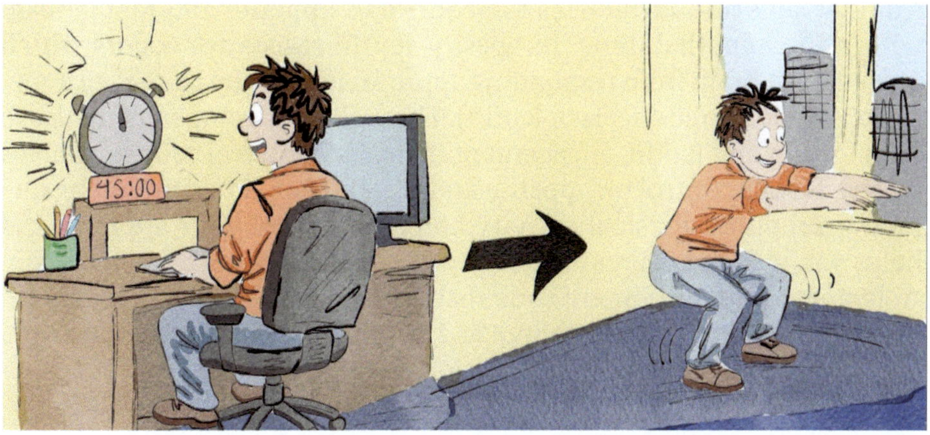

Figure 7.3: Converting 'bibuttockism' to punctuated sedentariness.

The Metabolic Benefits of Physical Activity

When we engage in physical exercise, or any physical activity for that matter, this sets in motion all kinds of physiological processes that occur within our body, all happening at the same (or roughly the same) time. The salutary health benefits of physical activity have been recognised since Hippocrates, but even today we lack full understanding and insight into the physiological mechanisms involved (7). However, in recent years, we have gained much understanding from both rodent- and human-based studies. Here, I summarise some of those key insights.

As alluded to, regular engagement in physical activity reduces our cardiovascular risk and improves our cardiorespiratory fitness (that in turn is a good predictor of mortality). The 'curvilinear' relationship between physical activity and risk of cardiovascular mortality reveals that those of us who engage in no or only minimal physical activity stand to gain the most cardiovascular benefit by engaging in mild-moderate levels of physical activity (7). When we engage in physical activity, we also improve our overall metabolic efficiency, including insulin sensitivity within cells, and the ability of our cells and tissues to take up glucose (sugar) from the blood and utilise it within our cells. Accordingly, physical activity improves our glucose and lipid handling, with a net result of reducing our risk of developing conditions like Type 2 Diabetes Mellitus (or improving our blood sugar control if we already have Diabetes Mellitus) and improving our lipid profile (levels of cholesterol in the blood). These metabolic improvements undoubtedly contribute towards the beneficial impact of physical activity on our overall cardiovascular risk. Importantly for our discussion (and for the theme of Chapter 12), when we engage in regular physical activity, we also improve our leptin sensitivity (8). (Leptin is an adipokine that is released from fat cells and influences the control of appetite and metabolism within the hypothalamus. In obesity, leptin resistance occurs which prevents the brain from responding appropriately to the beneficial appetitive and metabolic effects of leptin). Through enhancing sensitivities to both insulin and leptin, engagement in regular physical activity enables more effective control of appetite and metabolism. Put simply, engagement in regular physical activity helps to control your appetite and helps you to avoid overeating. This process also improves metabolism. A 'leptogenic' environment (one that enables and facilitates increased engagement in physical activity), as I discuss in Chapter 12, is also one that enables leptin to do its proper job.

Beyond these benefits of improved cardiorespiratory fitness, appetite control, metabolic efficiency and cardiovascular risk, regular physical activity also improves the functioning of our fat tissue. Although the human-based studies are contentious, rodent-based studies suggest that white adipose tissue (the type that stores energy) can become 'beige' in response to physical activity and burn off more calories in the process (7). The science of this process is a bit complex, but essentially what this means is that less energy is stored and more energy is burnt off in the fat tissue and released as heat. In other words, regular physical activity improves our thermogenic potential. This is certainly true in humans when it comes to the improvement of SM mass and functioning that stems from regular physical activity, with optimisation of our metabolic rate in a way that is entirely healthy and will not put us at risk of hyperthermia.

You may be wondering what is going on from a physiological perspective when we engage in physical activity. To understand this, we need to introduce another term: 'exerkines'. These are small molecular metabolites that are released from diverse tissues during physical activity (exercise), including the SM (myokines), fat tissue (adipokines), liver (hepatokines) and bone (osteokines). These molecules have effects not only on distant organs and tissues but also on adjacent tissues (such as SM and fat tissue) and may even act on their own tissue of origin (*fig 7.4*). These exerkines, like 'irisin' (a myokine released from the SM during physical exercise), likely mediate multiple metabolic benefits of physical activity (7).

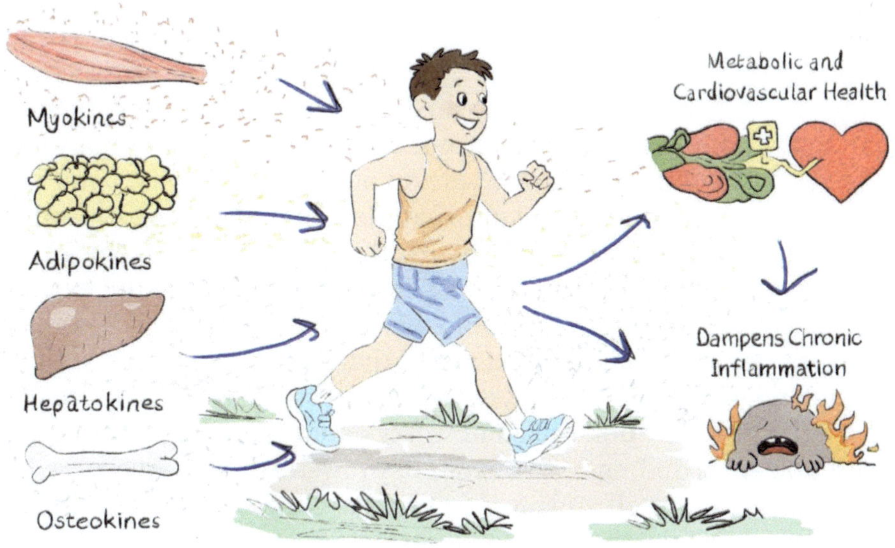

Figure 7.4: Thank exercise for exerkines.

We are not finished yet though, as regular physical activity also reduces chronic inflammation (a forerunner to Cardiovascular disease [CVD] and multiple other pathologies) through mechanisms that implicate exerkines (myokines like Interleukin-6, IL-6), that dampen the inflammatory cascade and improve body composition (reduced fat mass and increased SM mass). Furthermore, regular physical exercise also results in beneficial changes to the structure and function of the cardiovascular system itself. This includes 'cardiac hypertrophy' that relates to increased thickness of the heart muscle, in a similar way to enhancing the thickness of your biceps muscle in response to weightlifting with your arms. It is important to highlight that 'left ventricular hypertrophy' can also be a sign of pathology (including high blood pressure or hypertension). In its pathological form, cardiac hypertrophy can lead to stiffening within the heart muscle wall that in turn impairs the ability of the heart to pump blood. Conversely, healthy cardiac hypertrophy that is induced by regular physical exercise associates with improved elasticity within the heart wall. What this means practically is that the heart can fill with blood more easily during diastole (between each systolic heartbeat). Relaxation of the cardiac ventricles ('lusitropy') is not just a passive process but a key determinant of cardiovascular efficiency that can be optimised by engagement in regular physical exercise (7).

At this point, I would just offer one word of caution. As with most things in life, moderation is key. Engaging in extreme amounts of physical exercise can be harmful to us. I am not a cardiologist, but my colleague told me that they have seen the odd patient who is otherwise entirely fit and well, but whose cardiac output (the ability to pump blood around the body) has become physically compromised through extreme physical exercise-induced cardiac hypertrophy (where the grossly hypertrophied heart muscle physically restricts the flow of blood from the heart to the body). Harmful exercise-induced cardiac hypertrophy is not to be confused with the healthy version outlined in the last paragraph, and to be fair this condition is unusual. Redolent of driving to Hull (for those readers not based in the UK, Hull is a lovely city in the UK but is out on a limb geographically), the development of harmful exercise-induced cardiac hypertrophy would take a huge amount of determined and sustained effort to get there, rather than being something (or in the case of Hull, somewhere) that you would just stumble upon by accident. Most of us probably don't need to worry about this unusual condition, unless you are spending most of your day physically working out, which you are probably not. If you are, just beware: Unless you are an elite athlete, maybe just take things a bit easier.

Finally, we come to one benefit of physical activity that is perhaps less well known and appreciated. As we age, the main tube that carries blood from the heart to supply the entire body, the aorta, becomes less flexible and more stiffened. Essentially, the aorta becomes less able to absorb and dissipate some of the mechanical energy propagated by the pumping left ventricle. This is unfortunate as it means that there are bigger swings of blood pressure hitting the peripheral organs (the highs of systole are higher, and the lows of diastole are lower). This is called 'pulse pressure', and it is very important. Increased pulse pressure that stems from stiffening of the aorta is an important contributor to CVD (including impaired kidney function). And yes, you've guessed it! Regular engagement in physical exercise helps to improve elasticity within the aorta, thereby improving pulse pressure and reducing the risk for vascular damage in the peripheral organs (7).

To summarise this section, the metabolic health benefits of physical exercise are legion. We haven't even considered some of the other benefits of physical activity that include, for example, reduced vulnerability to the development of mental health problems (9). In short, our whole health and well-being depend upon us being physically active. There are, of course, aspects of exercise science that we do not yet fully understand. There is some heterogeneity in the response of individuals to physical activity and exercise. Furthermore, there may be some heterogeneity between individuals regarding the beneficial metabolic responses to physical activity and exercise based on its type and intensity. These unknowns are research questions for the future. However, our current knowledge and insights point towards one overarching learning point for most of us who are not elite athletes: engage more in physical activity! It is no exaggeration to say that your life depends on it.

How to Optimise Our Physical Activity

To conclude this chapter, we need to consider how we can all improve our physical activity in our daily lives. The first thing to highlight here is that when it comes to advice on physical activity, as with diet, we are all individuals, and it cannot be too prescriptive. When I see patients in my obesity clinic, there are a myriad of reasons that can stymie any attempt at increased physical activity. This may include physical limitations, knee, hip or back pains, reduced SM strength or breathlessness from the effort of moving and/or cardiovascular compromise. Then there are the feelings of embarrassment that can arise, promulgated by our cruel society in which obesity is stigmatised, predisposing people to make hurtful and abusive comments. Beyond these physical and societal hurdles, there are mental, emotional and motivational challenges. When you have a low mood, or you have had a bad day, or you simply have reduced energy levels, it can be difficult to find motivation to engage in physical activity. Finally, there are time limitations: finding the time in our busy lives to incorporate physical activities can be challenging.

As with the government 'one-size-fits-all' approach to diet, with its obsession and fixation on calories (discussed in Chapter 11), so too I think the government advice on physical exercise is too prescriptive and inflexible. This advises that as adults, we should aim for at least 150-minutes of moderate-intensity or 75-minutes of vigorous-intensity activity per week along with muscle-strengthening activities at least two days a week. This is all well and good, but many of us would struggle to achieve this ideal for all the reasons given above, and a million more. The problem is that having such 'one-size-fits-all' idealised and inflexible government guidance on physical exercise can have a demotivating effect on those who simply can't achieve it. This can then lead to people giving up on any form of physical activity with associated increased sedentariness. Although offered with good intentions, such official governmental advice may be doing more harm than good.

Faced with inflexible government advice and a myriad of factors that thwart our attempts to improve our engagement in physical activities, what can we do? This will vary for each of us, and it is important that you align your own approach to what is best for you. Don't compare yourself today with the elite athlete who may live next door to you. Rather, compare how your own personal physical activity is today compared with how it was yesterday for you and aim for your own personal improvement, progressively day on day. Here are some generic tips to help you on that journey:

- We live in a sick society in which obesity is stigmatised. If someone hurls abuse towards you whilst you are exercising, take comfort in the knowledge and insight that the person hurling the abuse, not you, has a problem. Their hurtful comment reveals more about them (and our wider society) than about you. Do not retaliate! The perpetrator will not feel better by behaving in this way, in fact the reverse. The reality is that in this scenario, you are improving your own future health outlook, and they are worsening theirs.
- If you do feel inhibited to engage in physical activities outside of your house or flat, then there are lots of physical activities that you can do inside. You don't need to necessarily invest in a home treadmill. As outlined earlier, squats are a good form of exercise!
- If you are able and motivated to engage in regular physical exercise of moderate or vigorous intensity, the kind that brings you out into a sweat, then that is excellent and will have all kinds of metabolic

benefits for you. However, if this is not possible for whatever reason(s), then it is very important that you still engage in regular physical activities, however light, with avoidance of prolonged uninterrupted sedentariness, as these measures will also provide all kinds of metabolic benefits for you.

- If you have a busy job, have childcare duties or care for a relative or other factors in your life that limit your time for formal engagement in physical exercise, then look at how you can incorporate more physical activities into your daily routine. It could be a simple measure like using the stairs rather than the lift at work, getting off the bus one stop earlier and walking more as a result. Whatever you do, and whoever you are, there will always be ways to improve your physical activity during the day. This is limited only by our imagination (and perhaps motivation too).
- Of course, when it comes to physical activity, we need to be sensible. There are people who have a seriously compromised cardiovascular system, in whom physical exercise is prohibitive. Be sensible and know your own limits. If you encounter any chest pain or other concerning symptoms whilst exercising, then obviously get it checked out by appropriately qualified healthcare professionals immediately.
- If you cannot mobilise or use your legs for whatever reason(s), then do not feel precluded from engaging in physical activity! There are multiple physical activities that involve arm movements, and this should be your focus. I know I said earlier that sedentariness is when we sit or lie in waking hours, but this is only generally true (as we are usually sedentary in those positions). However, this statement is not true in every scenario: we can use our SMs and be physically active when sitting and even when lying when doing the luge (or certain forms of yoga, perhaps).
- Perhaps the simplest way to reduce sedentariness is to stand up. Consider what measures could improve your standing time, like use of standing desks, for example.
- Do not underestimate walking as an excellent form of exercise. We evolved as a bipedal species, with walking as our main form of locomotion. We have genetic endowment to walk, and habitual (obligate) bipedal walking is a uniquely human activity.
- Finally, if you can, try to enjoy physical activity. If it helps, do it in pairs or a group to improve social interaction. This can also help with motivation. As a long-term strategy, any lifestyle intervention needs to be enjoyable. If running on a treadmill isn't your thing, then choose something that is.

References

1. Hanson P, Weickert MO, Barber TM. Obesity: novel and unusual predisposing factors. Ther Adv Endocrinol Metab. 2020;11:2042018820922018.
2. Melanson EL. The effect of exercise on non-exercise physical activity and sedentary behavior in adults. Obes Rev. 2017;18(Suppl 1):40–9.
3. Pontzer H, Durazo-Arvizu R, Dugas LR, Plange-Rhule J, Bovet P, Forrester TE, et al. Constrained total energy expenditure and metabolic adaptation to physical activity in adult humans. Curr Biol. 2016;26(3):410–7.
4. Vallance JK, Gardiner PA, Lynch BM, D'Silva A, Boyle T, Taylor LM, et al. Evaluating the evidence on sitting, smoking, and health: is sitting really the new smoking? Am J Public Health. 2018;108(11):1478–82.
5. Gao Y, Li QY, Finni T, Pesola AJ. Enhanced muscle activity during interrupted sitting improves glycemic control in overweight and obese men. Scand J Med Sci Sports. 2024;34(4):e14628.
6. Diniz DG, Bento-Torres J, da Costa VO, Carvalho JPR, Tomas AM, Galdino de Oliveira TC, et al. The hidden dangers of sedentary living: insights into molecular, cellular, and systemic mechanisms. Int J Mol Sci. 2024;25(19):10757.
7. Belanger MJ, Rao P, Robbins JM. Exercise, physical activity, and cardiometabolic health: pathophysiologic insights. Cardiol Rev. 2022;30(3):134–44.
8. Fontana A, Vieira JG, Vianna JM, Bichowska M, Krzysztofik M, Wilk M, et al. Reduction of leptin levels during acute exercise is dependent on fasting but not on caloric restriction during chronic exercise: a systematic review and meta-analysis. PLoS One. 2023;18(11):e0288730.
9. Rodriguez-Romo G, Acebes-Sanchez J, Garcia-Merino S, Garrido-Munoz M, Blanco-Garcia C, Diez-Vega I. Physical activity and mental health in undergraduate students. Int J Environ Res Public Health. 2022;20(1):195.

8 Fibre: A Forgotten Dietary Macronutrient

'Beans, beans, they're good for your heart. The more you eat, the more you...' Yes, well that is enough of that! We can recall as children having a good laugh at this little ditty describing one of the nation's favourite foods. As adults, we may still have a laugh about it with our own children. Beans are an excellent example of a food packed full of dietary fibre, the focus of this chapter. Whoever first penned this aphorism was prescient. As it turns out, beans and other sources of dietary fibre are indeed good for your heart and have a whole load of other health benefits besides. Beans are also an excellent nutrient source for our gut microbiota that we discussed in Chapter 5. This explains the second part of the aphorism and one potential limitation of a high-fibre diet. Our interest in dietary fibre goes back over 2,000 years with Hippocrates who first described the laxative effects of coarse wheat (1). In the 1920s, publications from Kellogg (yes, the name behind some of our cereals), outlined some of the health benefits of bran (including 'laxation' and stool weight) (1, 2). In 2020, I published a scientific review article on the health benefits of dietary fibre in the journal, *Nutrients* (3). At the time of writing, this paper now has >1,100 citations and has become my most highly cited paper and one of the most highly cited papers in recent times in the field of dietary fibre research. Whilst writing this chapter, I gave an interview for '*BBC Food*' on the health benefits of dietary fibre (`https://www.bbc.co.uk/food/articles/fibremaxxing`). This interview was sparked by a trend in social media circles advocating a high-fibre diet. Despite all the phoney fad diets and trends out there, this one is spot on, and I would like to think that this trend was influenced in some way by my own published review article.

Whilst I was growing up and for much of the last half century, there has been an inordinate amount of focus on dietary fat and how to limit this through a 'low-fat' diet (4). Interestingly, the whole 'low-fat' mindset which predominated in the latter half of the 20th century, stemmed from an attempt by the physicians of President Eisenhower to prevent his premature death from Cardiovascular disease (CVD). These 'insights' based on selective (and quite possibly biased) global epidemiological data became accepted dietary wisdom in the Western world. In this context, fat is the 'bad boy' of dietary nutrients based on its high caloric load. This is unfortunate given that there are examples of healthy forms of fat, such as polyunsaturated and monounsaturated fats, that we need for a healthy diet. I suspect that one reason for fat having such a bad name is precisely because of its name. Shakespeare famously asked, 'what's in a name?' When it comes to our diet and our understanding of the healthiness of the nutrients that we eat, the answer it seems is quite a lot! We use the term 'fat' as a pejorative descriptor for obesity. It is natural therefore for us to assume that by eating fat, this makes us fat! This is a simplistic way of thinking though. If anything, the excessive sugar content of ultra-processed foods (UPFs) is a greater contributor to weight gain and obesity than dietary fat (excessive sugar is converted to fat in the liver, that is then stored in the fat tissue, and may get deposited ectopically in the liver, skeletal muscles and heart and contribute towards conditions like Type 2 Diabetes Mellitus [T2D] and CVD). More recently, there has been a shift of focus towards a 'low-carbohydrate' diet (5), with examples of 'sugar taxes' and limitations on food advertising for children. These policies are welcome.

With all this hullabaloo around the two biggies, dietary fat and sugar, we have left another dietary macronutrient in the wings, ignored and lurking in the shadows. We have been so focused on fat and sugar that we seem to have forgotten the essential health benefits of this poor forlorn macronutrient. Would dietary fibre please enter the stage? Now is your time in the limelight.

Dietary Fibre: What Is It?

Before delving into the health benefits of dietary fibre, we need to define what it is. It may surprise you to learn that dietary fibre is a form of carbohydrate. As a group, carbohydrates are remarkably heterogeneous. They are all made of single units (monomers: think of each monomer as a single LEGO brick). Carbohydrates can exist as just one or two monomers, and these are broken down and digested easily and commonly known as sugar (for example, table sugar, sucrose, is formed of just two carbohydrate monomers [glucose and fructose] and so is easily broken down in the gut and absorbed). Carbohydrates can also exist as long strands of monomers. When these strands exceed around 10 monomers (so-called polysaccharides: think of 10 bricks stacked on top of one another), they become difficult to digest in the gut (1). This is what dietary fibre is: long strands of carbohydrate monomers that the gut is unable to digest properly (*fig 8.1*). It is a little bit more complex than this, and the European Food Safety Authority (EFSA) provides a long list of

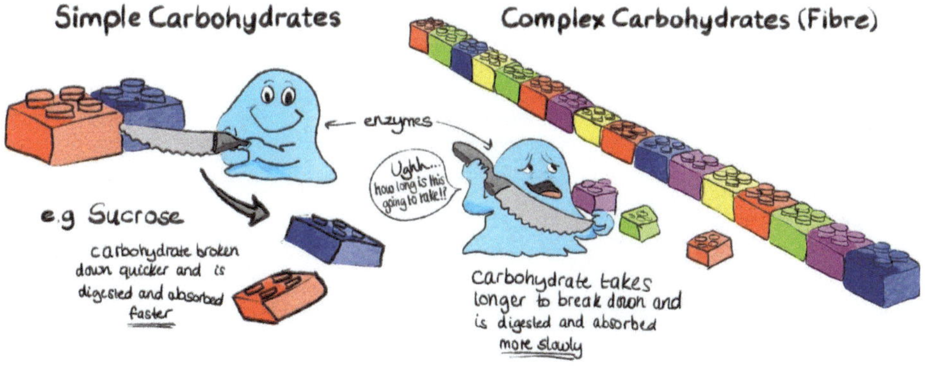

Figure 8.1: The quiddity of dietary fibre.

molecules that also constitute dietary fibre, including lignin, cellulose and pectins (1). Furthermore, although we may think of dietary fibre as being insoluble, there are soluble forms also that contribute towards health benefits. Dietary fibre is just long strands of carbohydrate monomers. Importantly, dietary fibre comes from plants, which is one of the reasons why a plant-based diet is healthy and why you often hear the promotion of plant-based foods as an integral part of a healthy diet.

Dietary Fibre: Why All the Fuss?

At this stage, you may be thinking about what all the fuss is about dietary fibre. Surely, we all get enough fibre from our diet. As it turns out, nothing could be further from the truth. In one of the largest reviews of dietary fibre intake in European populations (from early childhood to older adulthood) reported in 2017, this was 18–24 g and 16–20 g per day for men and women, respectively (6). Intake of dietary fibre was similar between countries and across age groups and higher than that in North American countries, based on data from the Nutrition Examination Survey (6). The current recommendations for dietary fibre intake in adults are 30–35 g and 25–32 g per day for men and women, respectively (6). It can be seen therefore that in Western countries, our dietary fibre intake is woefully inadequate and falls short by around one third of the recommended amount (*fig 8.2*). In other words, in Western countries, we should increase our intake of dietary fibre by around 50% (3).

Dietary Fibre: The Health Benefits

Over the last few decades, there has been a transformation in our understanding of the health benefits of dietary fibre. We now have data from multiple epidemiological studies that have been instrumental in

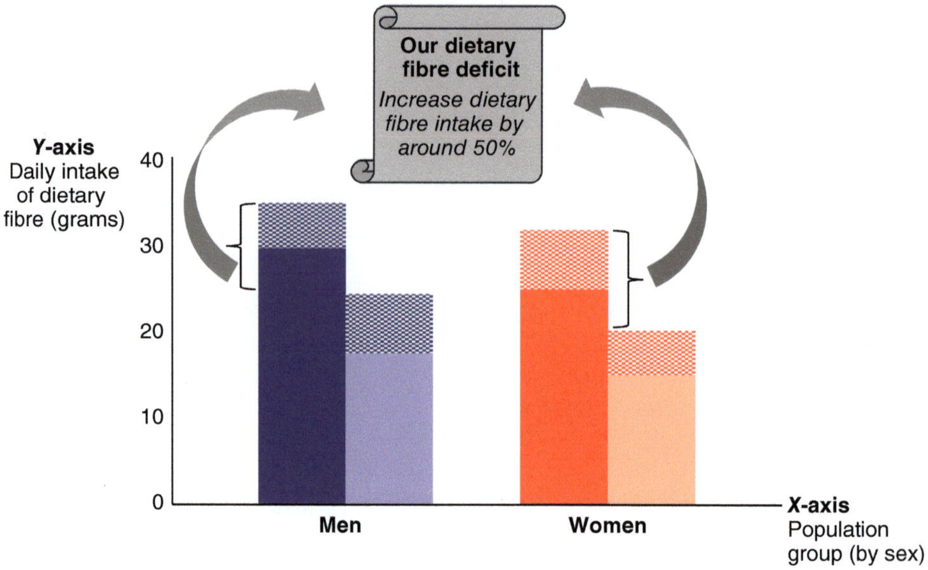

Figure 8.2: Our impoverishment of dietary fibre. The bars represent average daily intake of dietary fibre for men and women in the Western world. Dark blue: recommended daily intake for men; Light blue: actual daily intake for men; Dark red: recommended daily intake for women; Light red: actual daily intake for women. Hashed areas of each bar represent the range of daily fibre intake for each group.

providing us with such insights. We will start with the health benefit that is most familiar to us, that of gut motility and the avoidance of constipation. This is supported by a study that confirmed the alleviation of constipation through the consumption of 'vege-powder' (a mixture of broccoli, chicory and whole grains) (7). The role of dietary fibre in the prevention of constipation was confirmed by a systematic review on the topic (8). It is certainly true therefore that dietary fibre helps to keep our bowel motions regular and in the prevention of constipation.

What may be less well known and appreciated though is that in addition to the avoidance of constipation, dietary fibre can also help us to avoid dying or at least delay death. In a larger meta-analysis that analysed data from seven prospective cohort studies, all-cause mortality was reduced by 11% for every 10 g per day increase in dietary fibre intake (9). Have a look at that sentence again. By just increasing our dietary intake of fibre-replete plant-based foods by a little bit each day, we can reduce our risk of dying by over 10%! That is incredible. These data were confirmed in a further meta-analysis of data from 15 prospective cohort studies that also revealed reduced mortality from both CVD and all cancers with increased dietary intake of fibre, with the magnitude of effect being similar to that outlined earlier (10). There are few simple lifestyle changes that have such a marked effect on mortality (with smoking cessation and the avoidance of sedentariness being others). We do need to remember that there are potential confounders to such 'association' studies, and it may be, for example, that there is an association of the adoption of a high-fibre diet with other healthy lifestyle behaviours and that these also contribute towards improved mortality (3). With this caveat in mind though, the adoption of a high-fibre diet would seem sensible to improve your longevity.

So much for constipation and death. What about the other health benefits of dietary fibre?

At the start of this chapter, I said that dietary fibre is good for your heart. And so it is. In a large systematic review and meta-analysis of the literature that included data from 22 prospective cohort studies, it was shown that the intake of dietary fibre has an inverse relationship with the risk of CVD, including coronary heart disease (CHD) (11). Put simply, for every increase of 7 g per day of dietary fibre intake, this lowered relative risk of heart disease by 9% (11). Conversely, and in stark contrast, dietary intake of UPFs (based on data from >100,000 adult participants over a time period that exceeded 5-years) increased the risk of CVD, CHD and stroke (12).

At this point, I can hear myself in that famous clip with John Cleese from *Monty Python's Life of Brian*. 'Right, well apart from the alleviation of constipation, the delaying of death, and the reduced risk of CVD and CHD, what has dietary fibre ever done for us?' Well as it happens, just as the Romans did, a whole lot more. Multiple modern-day diseases have at their core, chronic inflammation. It is important to point out that this is not necessarily like having a grossly swollen knee or swollen tonsils, the kinds of inflammation that we may be familiar with. Rather, the chronic inflammation that I refer to here is much more insidious and hidden away within our tissues, and we will likely not even be aware of it. This is often a generalised process involving our peripheral tissues like fat depots and is important as it contributes towards multiple diseases, with T2D being just one example. It turns out that a diet that is impoverished of fibre is an important risk factor for the development of chronic inflammation (13, 14). Evidence for such an association includes data from overweight Hispanic and African-American adolescents, in which those who consumed high amounts of dietary fibre had substantially lower plasma markers of inflammation than those who consumed low amounts of dietary fibre (15). In a study on nearly 7,000 participants ('Airwave Health Monitoring Study'), there was a similar association between dietary fibre intake and improved inflammatory status, mediated partly by changes in body composition (16). Furthermore, dietary fibre supplements have been shown to improve inflammatory markers, albeit contingent on obesity status (17). Indirectly, the anti-inflammatory effects of dietary fibre may even alter the concentrations of neurotransmitters in the brain that could reduce the risk for the development of depression (18).

'Right, well apart from the alleviation of constipation, the delaying of death, the reduced risk of CVD and CHD, reduced chronic inflammation, and reduced risk of depression...' Dietary fibre also reduces our risk of developing certain cancers, most notably colorectal (or bowel) cancer, which is the third most common cancer globally. In a large systematic review and meta-analysis of the literature, dietary fibre reduced the risk of developing colorectal cancer by 26% (19). There is good evidence that dietary fibre improves our insulin sensitivity, which is important to protect us from the development of T2D and other dysmetabolic conditions (3). There is even evidence that a high-fibre diet may help us to lose weight, although admittedly the data for this are less compelling (3).

To summarise this section, the scientific evidence to support health benefits of dietary fibre is overwhelming. As intimated at the start of this chapter, these health benefits are not just restricted to being good for the heart, but extend to improving longevity, reducing risk of CVD and malignancies (that account for the majority of premature deaths in the Western world), putting a brake on inflammatory processes that underlies the pathophysiology of so many modern-day chronic diseases, reducing our risk of developing T2D and even protecting us from becoming depressed (*fig 8.3*). I mean, how much more evidence do we need? Surely, you may be thinking, it would be important for us all to consume plentiful dietary fibre, and this would be a great public health strategy to improve the health of the nation. Surely there should be improved awareness of the health benefits of dietary fibre, and our food should be replete with this most beneficial and yet somehow forgotten macronutrient. I will address these questions at the end of the chapter. Before that, let's consider how dietary fibre works.

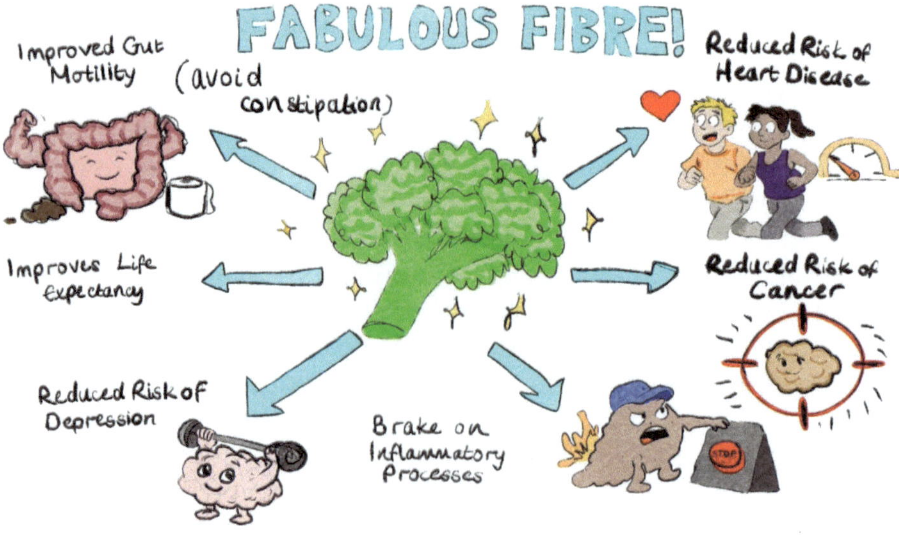

Figure 8.3: The health benefits of dietary fibre.

Dietary Fibre: How Does It Work?

In Chapter 5, I discussed the gut microbiota and its role in the maintenance of health and well-being and its importance in the context of the management of obesity. There are multiple aspects of our lifestyle that influence the composition of our gut microbiota. However, what is incontrovertible is the role of our diet. Dietary fibre is particularly important for our gut microbiota. There are multiple reasons. One useful analogy is the use of compost to fertilise the plants in our garden. In the same way, dietary fibre nurtures our gut microbiota. Importantly, our gut microbiota needs a food source, and dietary fibre provides this. Without a supply of dietary fibre, our gut microbiota uses an alternate food source, one produced by us, the sugary molecules present within our colonic mucus that provides a lining for the gut wall (20). 'So what?', I hear you ask. The problem with this is that our colonic mucus provides an essential defensive physical barrier between our gut microbiota and the lining of our gut (the 'colonic epithelium' or wall). When this mucus layer becomes depleted and breached (by the munching of fibre-impoverished gut microbiota), it leaves the lining of our gut wall exposed to attack by our gut microbiota. This can provoke an inflammatory reaction (colitis) and result in a 'leaky gut' in which parts of the gut microbiota migrate across the colonic wall into the blood and can then promote a chronic inflammatory reaction within the peripheral tissues (termed 'endotoxaemia'). This increases the risk of development of T2D and other chronic diseases.

Through its nurturing effect, dietary fibre also helps in the establishment and maintenance of diversity within our gut microbiota, which is so important for the state of eubiosis (referring to a healthy gut microbiota). We know that effective weight loss results in improved diversity within the gut microbiota (21) and therefore should represent an important goal in any management strategy for obesity. In addition to diversity within the gut microbiota, dietary fibre also enables our gut microbiota to produce 'metabolites' (molecules that are the by-products of metabolism) like 'short-chain fatty acids' (SCFAs). SCFAs have multiple health benefits, including the provision of an energy source (and therefore protection) for the cells in our gut wall ('colonocytes'), to improve the efficiency of metabolism of sugars and fats in the body and to regulate our appetite and control of metabolism (22). Conversely, a fibre-impoverished diet promotes restricted diversity within the gut microbiota, a state of dysbiosis. This has negative effects on the healthiness of our gut wall, the control of our appetite and metabolism, metabolic processing of essential nutrients, inflammatory processes and insulin sensitivity and therefore represents an important risk for the development of T2D and other chronic ill health (*fig 8.4*).

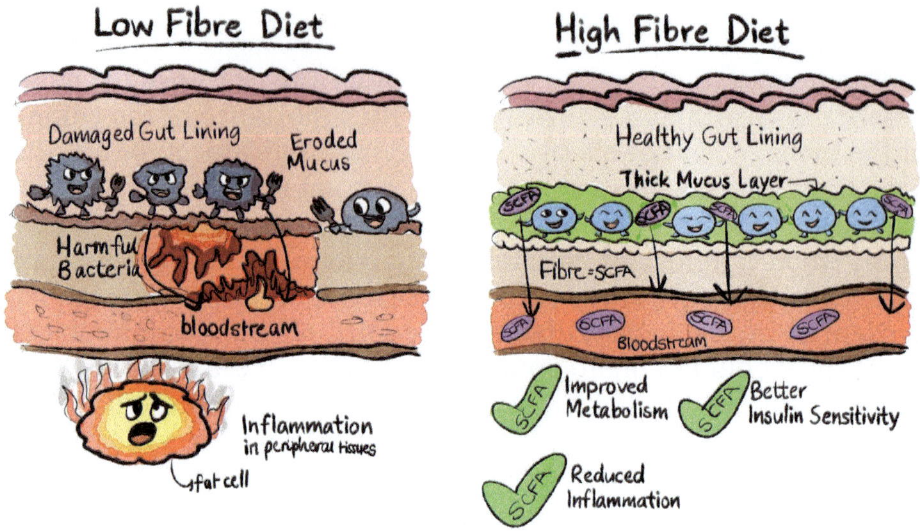

Figure 8.4: Dietary fibre in action.

It is fair to say that we don't fully understand how dietary fibre improves our health. There may be other mechanisms that do not implicate our gut microbiota. Furthermore, our insights with regards to the gut microbiota and their effects on health stem partly from rodent-based studies. However, based on our current understanding and insights, dietary fibre derived from plant-based foods plays an essential role in the establishment and nurture of a healthy gut microbiota that in turn helps to promote our own health and well-being (3).

Dietary Fibre: How to Optimise Our Intake?

By this stage, I hope that I have convinced you of the importance of a fibre-replete diet. Our health and well-being are dependent on it. If I have not convinced you, then frankly, I am not sure what will. However, it is one thing to be convinced by the data and quite another to incorporate this into our daily lives. (There are multiple examples of healthy lifestyle practices that are not widely adopted, not through lack of data, knowledge or understanding, but due to a multitude of other limiting factors). In Chapter 11, I discuss diet, and in Chapter 12, environmental factors that are relevant for our health and well-being, including our food environment. Here, I focus on how we can, as a population, improve our intake of dietary fibre, and how to address the factors that can hinder this approach.

Compared to the pre-industrialised era, our Western diets have changed radically. Our once fibre-replete diet, packed full of unprocessed plant-based foods, has been replaced by a diet predominated by UPFs (3). This scenario manifests a double whammy on our metabolic health, with an over-consumption of harmful sugars, saturated and trans fats and sodium (salt) and a deficit of dietary fibre (23). In the United Kingdom, most of our caloric intake (around 57%) comes from the intake of UPFs, with under a third (around 30%) from unprocessed (mainly plant-based) foods (23).

There are three main strategies that we can adopt to improve our intake of dietary fibre. The first is to improve the availability of high-fibre foods. Supermarket shopping has become the norm in Western societies. The food available to us in supermarkets influences what we eat. A common experience is that healthy fruit and vegetables occupy a small area of the typical Western supermarket, with the rest devoted to processed foods, including UPFs. One solution would be to redress this imbalance and provide a greater provision of unprocessed plant-based foods in our supermarkets, to replace a proportion of the shelving currently devoted to UPFs. Other approaches could be to facilitate, encourage and incentivise the re-emergence of greengrocers onto our high street. This was a common sight in our pre-supermarket era.

The second strategy is to ensure the widespread and ubiquitous manufacture of high-fibre food. For this, we need food companies to act more responsibly and for governments to legislate. In short, we need to ensure that our processed foods have added fibre that could replace harmful sugar and fats. One option would be for the addition of powdered broccoli, chicory or whole grains to certain foods (7). Whilst this may not appeal to all of us, it would at least be useful for consumers to have a choice of a healthier, fibre-replete version of processed food products. There would be substantial population-wide health benefits from adopting such an approach.

The third strategy requires cultural and societal changes. This includes changing our collective mindset with regards to high-fibre foods. The trend on social media alluded to at the start of this chapter is an excellent development. We could be more imaginative in our recipes that include fibre and maybe utilise a special app on our electronic devices that helps us to track our dietary fibre intake and encourages us to eat more fibre every day, analogous to how 'fitness-trackers' track our physical activity. Concurrently, we need to address the limitations of widespread adoption of a high-fibre diet. The clue is in the second part of the little aphorism that starts this chapter. A by-product of dietary fibre-induced diversity of the gut microbiota is the production of intestinal gas with its attendant unfortunate and sometimes embarrassing consequences. This can also lead to abdominal bloating and discomfort. Other people may struggle with the taste, appearance and digestibility of certain fibre-rich foods (3). Then we come to cost limitations. Unfortunately, healthy diets that are replete with fibre typically cost around 25–30% more than unhealthy UPF-based diets (3).

This leads to terrible inequalities within our population, in which those poorer members of society who are more likely to suffer from unhealthy lifestyles, weight gain and obesity are also those who would struggle most to afford a healthy fibre-replete diet. Governments should intervene to address these inequalities, with subsidies for healthy fibre-replete foods, particularly for those poorer members of our society. This would be the antithesis of (and indeed would complement) a sugar tax and would encourage and facilitate more of us to adopt a healthy diet.

There are multiple examples of how our lives have changed radically since the Industrial Revolution, with advances in technologies, agriculture, transport, medicines and education. (I can feel another *Monty Python* sketch coming on!) I find it incredible to think that whilst our lives have improved in so many ways, our diets have deteriorated and taken such a nosedive. Admittedly, this decline has played out primarily over the last 50-years, turbo-charged by the rise of UPFs in the 1980s, concurrent with the rise of supermarket culture. This scenario is remarkable given how important our diet is for our health and well-being. Of all the macronutrients to discuss, I have chosen to devote an entire chapter to dietary fibre. There are two main reasons for this. The first, as intimated earlier, is that there has been a near total eclipse of this essential macronutrient by its two big brothers (or sisters), sugar and fat, which have enjoyed the limelight over many decades. The second is the vast evidence base that supports the health benefits of dietary fibre and a population-wide lack of awareness of these benefits beyond the alleviation of constipation.

So come out from the gloomy wings and enter the stage, dietary fibre. Now is your well-deserved time in the limelight. And for the sake of our future health and well-being, I hope that everyone enjoys and internalises the spectacular show that you provide (*fig 8.5*).

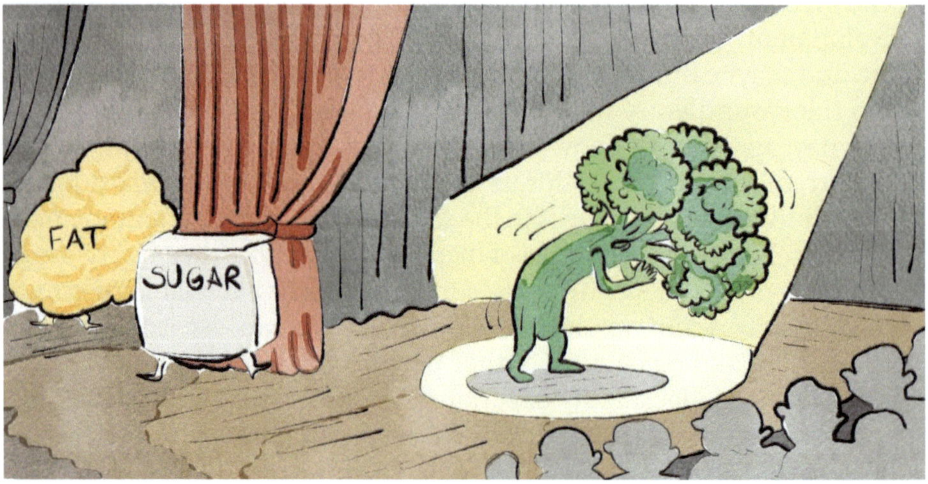

Figure 8.5: Dietary fibre, take a bow.

And with that, it is time for my dinner. I feel like broccoli tonight….

References

1. Hijova E, Bertkova I, Stofilova J. Dietary fibre as prebiotics in nutrition. Cent Eur J Public Health. 2019;27(3):251–5.
2. Slavin JL. Dietary fiber: classification, chemical analyses, and food sources. J Am Diet Assoc. 1987;87(9):1164–71.
3. Barber TM, Kabisch S, Pfeiffer AFH, Weickert MO. The health benefits of dietary fibre. Nutrients. 2020;12(10):3209.
4. Harcombe Z. Dietary fat guidelines have no evidence base: where next for public health nutritional advice? Br J Sports Med. 2017;51(10):769–74.
5. Hinde S. Understanding the role of carbohydrates in optimal nutrition. Nurs Stand. 2019;34(8):76–82.
6. Stephen AM, Champ MM, Cloran SJ, Fleith M, van Lieshout L, Mejborn H, et al. Dietary fibre in Europe: current state of knowledge on definitions, sources, recommendations, intakes and relationships to health. Nutr Res Rev. 2017;30(2):149–90.
7. Woo HI, Kwak SH, Lee Y, Choi JH, Cho YM, Om AS. A controlled, randomized, double-blind trial to evaluate the effect of vegetables and whole grain powder that is rich in dietary fibers on bowel functions and defecation in constipated young adults. J Cancer Prev. 2015;20(1):64–9.
8. Rao SS, Yu S, Fedewa A. Systematic review: dietary fibre and FODMAP-restricted diet in the management of constipation and irritable bowel syndrome. Aliment Pharmacol Ther. 2015;41(12):1256–70.
9. Kim Y, Je Y. Dietary fiber intake and total mortality: a meta-analysis of prospective cohort studies. Am J Epidemiol. 2014;180(6):565–73.
10. Kim Y, Je Y. Dietary fibre intake and mortality from cardiovascular disease and all cancers: a meta-analysis of prospective cohort studies. Arch Cardiovasc Dis. 2016;109(1):39–54.
11. Threapleton DE, Greenwood DC, Evans CE, Cleghorn CL, Nykjaer C, Woodhead C, et al. Dietary fibre intake and risk of cardiovascular disease: systematic review and meta-analysis. BMJ. 2013;347:f6879.
12. Srour B, Fezeu LK, Kesse-Guyot E, Alles B, Mejean C, Andrianasolo RM, et al. Ultra-processed food intake and risk of cardiovascular disease: prospective cohort study (NutriNet-Sante). BMJ. 2019;365:l1451.
13. Bach Knudsen KE, Laerke HN, Hedemann MS, Nielsen TS, Ingerslev AK, Gundelund Nielsen DS, et al. Impact of diet-modulated butyrate production on intestinal barrier function and inflammation. Nutrients. 2018;10(10):1499.
14. Gogebakan O, Kohl A, Osterhoff MA, van Baak MA, Jebb SA, Papadaki A, et al. Effects of weight loss and long-term weight maintenance with diets varying in protein and glycemic index on cardiovascular risk factors: the diet, obesity, and genes (DiOGenes) study: a randomized, controlled trial. Circulation. 2011;124(25):2829–38.
15. Miller SJ, Batra AK, Shearrer GE, House BT, Cook LT, Pont SJ, et al. Dietary fibre linked to decreased inflammation in overweight minority youth. Pediatr Obes. 2016;11(1):33–9.

16. Gibson R, Eriksen R, Chambers E, Gao H, Aresu M, Heard A, et al. Intakes and food sources of dietary fibre and their associations with measures of body composition and inflammation in UK adults: cross-sectional analysis of the Airwave Health Monitoring Study. Nutrients. 2019;11(8):1839.
17. Kabisch S, Meyer NMT, Honsek C, Gerbracht C, Dambeck U, Kemper M, et al. Obesity does not modulate the glycometabolic benefit of insoluble cereal fibre in subjects with prediabetes—a stratified post hoc analysis of the Optimal Fibre Trial (OptiFiT). Nutrients. 2019;11(11):2726.
18. Swann OG, Kilpatrick M, Breslin M, Oddy WH. Dietary fiber and its associations with depression and inflammation. Nutr Rev. 2020;78(5):394–411.
19. Gianfredi V, Salvatori T, Villarini M, Moretti M, Nucci D, Realdon S. Is dietary fibre truly protective against colon cancer? A systematic review and meta-analysis. Int J Food Sci Nutr. 2018;69(8):904–15.
20. Desai MS, Seekatz AM, Koropatkin NM, Kamada N, Hickey CA, Wolter M, et al. A dietary fiber-deprived gut microbiota degrades the colonic mucus barrier and enhances pathogen susceptibility. Cell. 2016;167(5):1339–53 e21.
21. Koutoukidis DA, Jebb SA, Zimmerman M, Otunla A, Henry JA, Ferrey A, et al. The association of weight loss with changes in the gut microbiota diversity, composition, and intestinal permeability: a systematic review and meta-analysis. Gut Microbes. 2022;14(1):2020068.
22. den Besten G, van Eunen K, Groen AK, Venema K, Reijngoud D-J, Bakker BM. The role of short-chain fatty acids in the interplay between diet, gut microbiota, and host energy metabolism. J Lipid Res. 2013;54(9):2325–40.
23. Rauber F, da Costa Louzada ML, Steele EM, Millett C, Monteiro CA, Levy RB. Ultra-processed food consumption and chronic non-communicable diseases-related dietary nutrient profile in the UK (2008(-)2014). Nutrients. 2018;10(5):587.

9

Listening

In the early 1980s, I attended Oxbridge Lane Primary School in Stockton-on-Tees. Whilst there, every Tuesday afternoon we would have a 'singalong'. (Nowadays, I spend my Tuesday afternoons seeing patients in one of my obesity clinics. I am passionate about improving the lives of people living with obesity, but I am also passionate about music, and enjoy singing.) One of the songs was about the rainbow. You probably know it: 'Red and yellow and pink and green...'. Anyway, I recall that one of the lines in the song is: 'Listen with your eyes'. As a young child at the time, these lyrics made no sense to me. I think I probably assumed that the word 'see' should have been used instead of 'listen', but that 'listen' was chosen as its disyllabic form fitted better with the rhythm of the music. Now, over 40 years on, these lyrics resonate with me.

To explore further what is meant by 'listen with your eyes', we need to take a step back. We all understand intuitively our primary senses. This is how we experience the external world, and without these senses our world would be a very lonely place indeed. Our senses connect us with the world and the people and things in it. We can see the colours of the rainbow, and we can hear birdsong and Handel's Messiah. We can also see and hear a million other things every day. Most of these signals are just 'noise'. To deal with this influx of incoming signals, the brain needs to be highly selective and filters out most of what we sense (the unimportant noisy signals). This protects our poor cerebral cortices from being overloaded and is extremely important for normal brain function.

Traditionally, we use the term 'listen' to refer to the auditory sense, the sound signals that reach our ears that we hear. Emphatically though, listening is different from hearing. We can hear Handel's Messiah, but to appreciate this glorious music, we need to really listen to it. What this means in practical terms is that we give the music our full attention and focus, without being distracted. In doing so, we can morph our mental state into that which becomes at one with the music. Psychologists sometimes call this state 'flow'. Anyone who has experienced flow will understand intuitively what it is and how it feels. Of course, flow is not just restricted to listening to music or even to focusing on any sensory input but can also relate to engagement in certain physical activities or even thinking itself. Flow is a state in which you are fully present and engrossed entirely in the here and now, in whatever activity you are doing and is usually a pleasurable experience. Effectively, flow represents a pinnacle or paragon of listening, and its achievement should be considered as a blessing.

As with flow, the art of listening is not restricted to music or even to the auditory sense. In this chapter, I use the word ‘listening’ as an umbrella term that essentially refers to any incoming signal reaching the brain. This includes not only signals originating from the primary senses but also, importantly, the signals that originate from within our brain (thoughts) and from our bodies that constantly update our brain to tell us how we are and alert us to any emergent problems. One could also include social signals on this list, that is, the social cues that we receive from others in our everyday lives. In this context, ‘listen with your eyes’ makes a lot more sense! Like any art, we all need to learn how to listen. This is not easy, especially if we are required to ‘listen’ to something that we don’t want to ‘hear’. Another problem is that as humans, our brain is very good at deceiving us. This is called ‘cognitive bias’. Have you ever noticed that if an outcome of something that is important to you doesn’t go your way, you and others will come up with reasons why you were better off without that outcome anyway? This is cognitive bias at play, and it has evolved presumably as a way of protecting us from the mental, physical and social sequelae and burden of unfavourable events and outcomes: a way of minimising the mental and emotional blow so to speak. Cognitive bias can impair our ability to listen, and it is important that we are aware of this. Cognitive bias aside, I believe that we have forgotten and lost the art of listening, and we are all suffering as a result.

In my lifetime, our modern-day world has changed radically. In fact, in centuries to come, our current age will probably be labelled as the ‘Information Revolution’ that followed on from the Industrial Revolution and Scientific and Agricultural Revolutions before that. Imagine what it must have been like for our ancestors living at the dawn of the Industrial Revolution, with weird mills appearing in the landscape, and chimneys with smoke billowing out of them and subsequently noisy and scary locomotives equipped with fires, steam and smoke chugging along tracks, occasionally setting fire to overhanging branches! Although perhaps not as visually dramatic regarding our built environment, I think the current Information Revolution that we are all bearing witness to is no less impactful on our lives. The term ‘revolution’ is apt given the magnitude with which all our lives have changed radically in the 21st century, with the rise of the internet, electronic personal devices and artificial intelligence. At the click of a button, we can now access pretty much any information we want. Information is accessible to us 24/7 in a way that would have been inconceivable just half a century ago when I was born. We are also all connected with each other and the world in ways that are unprecedented in human history: the world has become a much smaller place. This quantum leap in information accessibility and connectiveness has and will continue to change the world and the human population radically.

So much for the Information Revolution. But what effect has this had on us? In our modern-day world, it seems that everyone should have an opinion. Social media encourages us to share these opinions with the outside world, and this is reinforced by 'likes' and other superficial indicators of approval. We are constantly bombarded with images and sounds from our electronic devices that follow us everywhere we go and vie for our attention. In fact, the success of each social media company depends, at least to some extent, on how much attention and 'airtime' it can gain from each of us, its users. This means that social media content tends to be selected for its ability to catch and hold our attention, rather than necessarily for its veracity or any other redeeming features that may ultimately benefit us. Our modern-day world seems to be defined by an emphasis on 'voice', and much of our lives seem to be about getting ourselves heard and putting in our own two pennyworth. But is anyone listening?

One problem with our modern-day world, with its emphasis on voice and opinion, bombardment with attention-grabbing images and sounds, our unprecedented access to information 24/7 and our connectedness to everyone and everything else, is that our brains have become overloaded (1). Unfortunately, this is a perfect storm to put a kibosh on the art of active listening. In fact, it could be said that our modern-day environment represents the antithesis of an environment that is conducive to active listening. Why should this be so? The reason is that to properly listen to anything or anyone, we need to focus on it, and with too many distractions this is simply not possible: we don't have enough brain power. Our brains need time and space to reflect and declutter and, crucially, time and space in which distractions are minimised. Only then can we truly be positioned to actively listen to anything or anyone. Buddhism seems to have understood this for millennia, with its quiet and decluttered environments, minimalist gardens and emphasis on meditation, for example.

That's a long preamble. You may, at this stage, be wondering why I am rambling on about stuff that seemingly has nothing to do with obesity! Nothing could be further from the truth. It turns out that our modern-day environment has a lot to do with obesity in many ways and not just the usual suspects of food- and diet-related reasons. You see, as I mentioned earlier, the brain is constantly being updated from the body by signals that alert it to any emergent problem or need. These are called 'interoceptive' signals. Think of the brain like a satellite orbiting the Earth, picking up 'pings' from Earth-related objects, the 'pings' being the interoceptive signals. It is a tragic metaphor, but one of the main reasons we know that flight MH370 ended up in the Indian Ocean is that it continued to send 'interoceptive' signals that were detected by an orbiting satellite. Had it not been for these signals and the listening satellite, the mystery of what happened to this flight would have been even greater. Most of the time, these interoceptive signals simply inform the brain that all is good, and are simply ignored. However, some signals, such as pain, send an alarm to the brain to act. Other signals, such as appetite, alert the brain to a particular need. Appetite is a special interoceptive signal for our discussion that I discussed in detail in Chapter 2. Although complex in its origins, appetite is something that we feel and can be thought of as a drive to eat food. It's the body's way of telling us that it is time to eat something, just like thirst drives us to drink fluid.

All this sounds very simple. The problem is that in our modern-day world, our brains are so distracted and overloaded that many of us have lost the ability to listen properly to our appetite and other interoceptive signals. The result? Well, many of us eat when we are not feeling hungry. In some scenarios, this could be 'mindless eating' in which food (often unhealthy snacks) is consumed subconsciously whilst engaging in some other activity. There are multiple other aspects of our modern-day world that compound the unfortunate distraction of our appetite. Firstly, eating is often a highly social activity. Food and eating often form an integral part of human group activities, events and celebrations (to be fair, this has probably always been the case). As humans, we are a highly social species, and it can be very hard not to eat (even when we don't feel hungry) when your social group are all eating (2). Have you ever noticed how compelled you feel to eat food from a buffet when everyone else in your group is eating from the same buffet? Furthermore, eating is usually a pleasurable experience. Many of us eat to experience the hedonic effects of food, to cheer ourselves up when we have had a bad day, if we feel low or even if we are just bored (3). Our modern-day culture and environment, with easy and readily available '24/7' access to (often unhealthy) food, have created a scenario in which we are enabled to eat almost at any time or place, for all kinds of reasons as outlined here, and not necessarily in response to our appetitive interoceptive signals. Finally, social media may also impact on our eating behaviour (4). The point I am trying to make here is that although appetite and hunger have evolved as a way of alerting our brain to eat, it seems like our modern-day environment has almost been designed in a way to effectively ignore and countermand these important bodily signals. Our ability to listen has become severely impaired (*fig 9.1*).

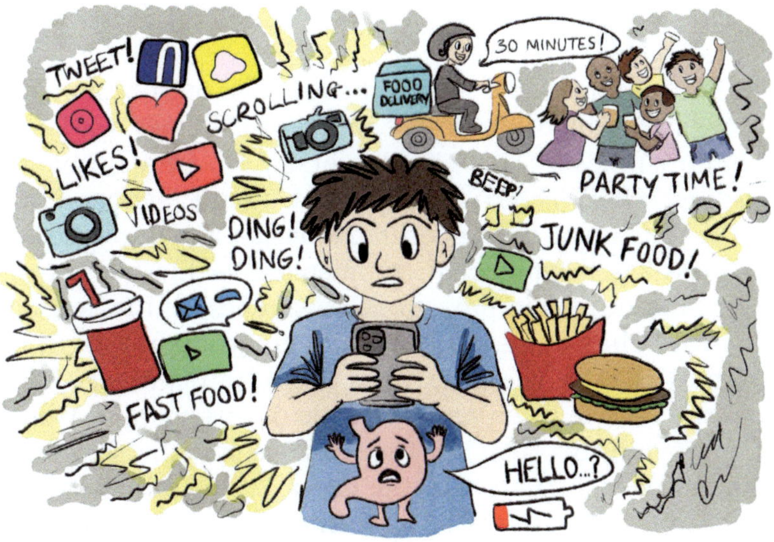

Figure 9.1: Our distracted modern-day world.

To be clear, I am not for one minute suggesting that we should only ever eat when we are hungry and that we should all lead ascetic lives, in which we avoid food at social occasions or even sometimes eating to cheer ourselves up when we might not feel hungry. We are humans, not machines. Like you, I enjoy a good buffet or barbeque with social groups and sometimes feel compelled to eat when I am not necessarily hungry. I also openly admit that, like many of us, I do sometimes eat to cheer myself up. I don't want this chapter to sound like I am preaching a message from some divine or 'holier-than-thou' standpoint. Being an obesity expert does not preclude me from being human and living in our modern-day environment! The key messages and learning points from this chapter I apply to myself as much as to anyone else. We need to enjoy our lives, and we need to be realistic. But I do think that we can all learn to listen more to our appetite and be more aware of our eating behaviours. Where possible, we should try to eat in response to hunger, as hard as this is at times. Our appetite evolved for a reason, and just as with any other interoceptive signal, we need to listen and respond to it appropriately and treat it with respect. In essence, we need to listen more to our appetite. This includes the habituated behaviour of eating 3 meals per day (breakfast, lunch and evening meal) that many of us adopt. We didn't evolve to eat 3 meals a day, and if we don't feel hungry, then we shouldn't feel compelled to eat 3 meals per day in a habitual manner. In fact, our physiology is better suited to some periods of relative caloric omission, to provide our liver with a break from being bombarded with nutrients (5). So, nothing bad is going to happen from occasionally missing a meal because we don't feel hungry, and this is probably a good thing for the body.

Since 2010, I have led a 'tier 3' hospital-based obesity service at the Warwickshire Institute for the Study of Diabetes, Endocrinology and Metabolism (WISDEM) at University Hospitals Coventry and Warwickshire (UHCW) NHS Trust in the United Kingdom. Within this service, I led a team of colleagues in the design and implementation of a mindfulness-based approach to complement the lifestyle management of obesity. Mindfulness improves one's awareness of the here and now, of one's own behaviour and immediate environment (both internal and external) at any given time. Does this sound familiar? In essence, mindfulness is active listening, the theme of this chapter. Mindfulness stems from Buddhism originally. There is great potential for mindfulness in all aspects of healthcare. For the naysayers who may be put off by the idea of mindfulness or who may think this is just another fad, my response would be to listen to and be guided by the evidence before formulating that opinion. We have demonstrated that the adoption of mindfulness within our tier 3 obesity service improves body weight and eating-related behaviours significantly (including avoiding 'mindless eating' when not feeling hungry, for example). We also showed that mindfulness improves the self-esteem and self-confidence of our patients. We published these data in a highly respected peer-reviewed journal (6). Based on this evidence, and further published research, our mindfulness approach culminating in our development and implementation of the 'W8 Buddy' lifestyle app (7), has even been recognised and endorsed by the National Institute for Health and Care Excellence (NICE) for use within tier 3 obesity-management centres throughout the National Health Service (NHS) in the United Kingdom.

How can we declutter our lives and enable ourselves to listen more to our body's interoceptive (including appetitive) signals? Just as with the Agricultural Revolution, the Information Revolution does seem irreversible, and we would not necessarily want to reverse it. We need to be realistic therefore and accept that we cannot change the world! However, each of us can make important changes. The first step is to recognise the problem and the need for us to listen more. It may help to make time and space each day for quiet and undistracted contemplation, to keep in tune with the body's interoceptive signals. This is an important step to facilitate active listening. In our modern-day world, many of us have increasing demands on our time, from our work, our relationships, our parental and caring duties and the like. At times, life can seem like a challenge in which the aim is to cram in as much as possible. The post COVID-19 era with the rise of virtual meetings has facilitated this, with the ability to have 'back-to-back' meetings, with no need for travel between each of them! Sometimes, we try to cram so much into our daily

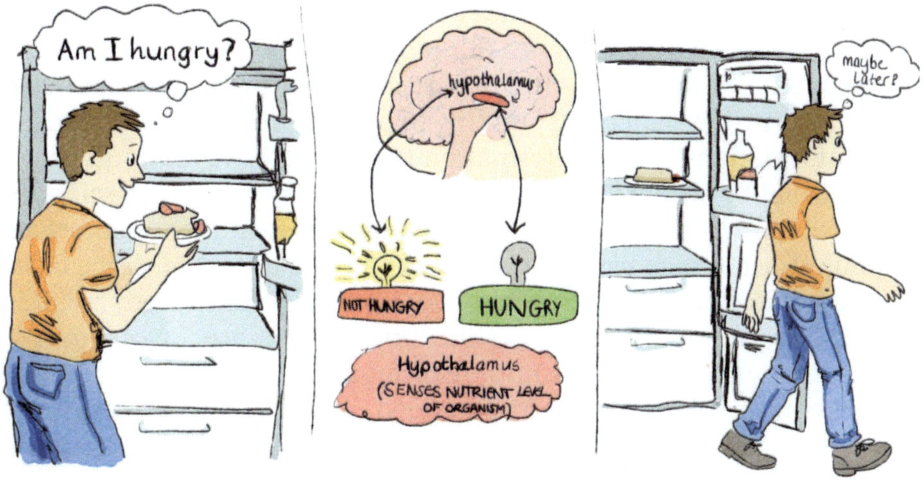

Figure 9.2: Listen to your appetite.

lives that even our sleep can be encroached upon, and devalued in the process. We need to recognise that this mindset is not healthy and conducive to active listening. Through allowing ourselves to listen more, this will ultimately improve our health and well-being and therefore enable us to be more productive in our lives in the longer term. Rather than trying to do more, we should utilise the mantra, 'less is more', and just slow down a bit. Before eating anything, ask yourself the question, 'Am I hungry?' If the answer is 'no', then consider not eating and putting back that bit of food from whence it came! (*fig 9.2*).

In addition to interoceptive signals from the body, we should also learn to listen more to the opinions of others. This includes experts. A while ago, I had an interview for an online tabloid newspaper in the United Kingdom, on the topic of obesity. Within hours of its publication, there were hundreds of comments from readers, each one published online for the world to read. I assume that these comments were not all from obesity experts. Whilst at times quite amusing to read, the comments often suggested a superiority of their opinion over all others, including mine. It is interesting that had I been an astrophysicist and provided the media with an expert opinion on something arcane and esoteric like the nature of dark matter, there probably would not have been too many non-experts who would have enlightened the world with their opinion on the matter. There may have been comments from a couple of 'flat-earther' types or conspiracy theorists. But with obesity, it sometimes seems like everyone is an expert. Why should this be? It is probably because obesity is personal to a large part of the populace. Within the United Kingdom, one in four adults live with obesity. The remaining 75% of adults will often know someone in their in- or out-groups who is living with obesity. Our own experiences that are personal to us, including what we see every day, influence our individual thoughts, opinions and beliefs about the world. This bias has a name: the 'availability heuristic'. Furthermore, there is a compounding of our personal bias by a tsunami of disinformation and misinformation that we all have ready access to, promulgated by non-experts and often without any supportive scientific evidence. Rather than allowing such distractions to influence ourselves, we should listen to experts and learn from their expertise. To be clear, I am not suggesting that expert opinion is infallible. Indeed, NICE in the United Kingdom considers expert opinion as the lowest form of clinical evidence. This does not mean that expert opinion is useless. Rather, correctly in my view, data derived from randomised controlled trials, or even better a meta-analysis of multiple randomised controlled trials, is superior to that of expert opinion. It is fine (indeed important) to question experts. But questioning requires us to listen to them first.

So go ahead, listen. Listen to your body's interoceptive signals and make time and space for this to happen. Listen to your appetite. Listen to the opinions of others, and don't assume that your opinion trumps that of everyone else! There may be important learning opportunities that can only be gained through listening, and of course active listening forms a foundation for good communication. Emphatically, listening is not the same as agreeing! Indeed, question everything, and then form your own opinion. A prerequisite though of intelligent questioning is active listening. Therefore, we need to learn to listen first and then question later. Be prepared to change your mind, and in this process, embrace humility. Rather than a sign of weakness, humility is, in my view, a sign of great strength. Indeed, humility is one of the greatest of all human attributes. Having the humility to change one's mind based on active listening and intelligent questioning is a sign of great strength. Be aware of the dangers of the Information Revolution, and that with this unprecedented and ready access to a universe of information, there is also ready access to a profusion of disinformation and misinformation that can distract, delude and discombobulate us. Listen to and learn from the experts. Listen to your senses. Indeed, listen with your eyes. And (as the song goes and if you feel so inclined), sing everything you see!

References

1. Barber TM, Kabisch S, Pfeiffer AFH, Weickert MO. Dietary and lifestyle strategies for obesity. Nutrients. 2024;16(16):2714.
2. Barberis N, Gugliandolo MC, Costa S, Cannavo M. Healthy and binge eating behaviours: the motivational processes underlying peer pressure. Psychol Health Med. 2022;27(5):1144–53.

3. Barrington WE, Beresford SAA. Eating occasions, obesity and related behaviors in working adults: does it matter when you snack? Nutrients. 2019;11(10):2320.
4. Chung A, Vieira D, Donley T, Tan N, Jean-Louis G, Kiely Gouley K, et al. Adolescent peer influence on eating behaviors via social media: scoping review. J Med Internet Res. 2021;23(6):e19697.
5. Vasim I, Majeed CN, DeBoer MD. Intermittent fasting and metabolic health. Nutrients. 2022;14:3, 631.
6. Hanson P, Shuttlewood E, Halder L, Shah N, Lam FT, Menon V, et al. Application of mindfulness in a tier 3 obesity service improves eating behavior and facilitates successful weight loss. J Clin Endocrinol Metab. 2019;104(3):793–800.
7. Hanson P, Abdelhameed F, Sahir M, Parsons N, Panesar A, de la Fosse M, et al. Evaluation of the digital support tool Gro Health W8Buddy as part of tier 3 weight management service: observational study. J Med Internet Res. 2025;16(27):e62661.

10 Pharmacotherapies and the Future of Obesity Management

Way back in 2010, I published a paper that highlighted the weight-loss effects of the 'Glucagon-Like Peptide-1' (GLP-1) class of therapies (today, commonly known as the 'skinny jabs'), and their potential use as an effective therapy for obesity (1). Back then, no one talked about 'skinny jabs', and our focus was mainly on the glycaemic (sugar-related) benefits of this class of drug for patients living with Type 2 Diabetes Mellitus (T2D). Today, the GLP-1 class of drugs are still used for their glycaemic benefits, but this therapeutic effect has been eclipsed somewhat by the unprecedented interest in their weight-loss effects.

This chapter is all about GLP-1 injections ('skinny jabs'). The first point to make is that 'skinny jab' is not a medical term. It is not a term that tends to be used within the medical fraternity. I have published many scientific papers in peer-reviewed journals on this topic, and in none of them did I refer to the term 'skinny jab'. If I had, my paper would probably have been rejected outright. So where did this term come from, and why am I using it here? The 'skinny jab' was coined by the media, and it seems to have stuck. Whenever we see any media piece on obesity, the term 'skinny jab' is often used. This book is written for everyone. Those of us outside of the medical world should be forgiven for thinking that 'skinny jab' is a bona fide medical term. Just like young children learning the correct noun for each new object in their world, so too as adults if we are exposed enough to a particular naming word, it will tend to stick. A bit like using 'Hoover' to refer to a 'vacuum cleaner'. Most of us recognise the term 'skinny jab', and that is the reason I have chosen to use this non-medical term here (and throughout other chapters).

In recent times, the media coverage of the GLP-1 injections ('skinny jabs') has been truly remarkable. I use 'media' here to include all forms of media, including the mass media and coverage on social media. Almost every day, it seems that coverage of the 'skinny jabs' crops up in the media somewhere and in some form. I have been qualified as a medical doctor since 1998, and in 27-years I have never witnessed such widespread interest in a single drug class. Not even statins come close. This unprecedented interest in the 'skinny jabs' tells us something fundamental about modern-day Homo sapiens, about our deep-seated desire to lose weight and possibly also about the inherent challenges of successful weight loss in our modern-day obesogenic environment.

This chapter is intended to improve our understanding of the GLP-1 injections ('skinny jabs'), to address common misconceptions and myths and to provide a well-needed reality check. To truly understand these therapies, we need to go right back to the start of this story and explore how we got to now. It is a fascinating story that encompasses key insights into gut physiology, monsters (really), and has become a cynosure for the whole world, attracting the interests of 'Big Pharma' and >200 biotechnology companies globally as a 'multi-billion dollar' industry.

In the Beginning, There Was the 'Incretin Effect'

Our story begins over a century ago. In the late 19th century, observational studies revealed something that later became known as the 'incretin effect'. In a nutshell, these early experiments involved a human participant ingesting a fixed amount of sugar, following which their blood sugar levels were monitored over the next few hours. As would be expected, following a meal there is a small rise in blood sugar levels, which then comes back down to baseline over around 1–2 hours. The experimenters then administered the same amount of sugar to the same human participants but this time as an infusion into a vein. What they observed was that, similar to the response to orally administered sugar, there was also a rise and subsequent fall to baseline in blood sugar levels in the 1–2 hours after the infusion, but the rise in blood sugar with the infused sugar load was greater and more pronounced than that with the orally administered sugar. Claude Bernard tried to explain this disparity through the effects of the liver taking up glucose during the first pass portal circulation when sugar is administered orally. Following the discovery of insulin in 1921, it was hypothesised that differences in insulin release following glucose administration either orally or into a vein would account for the differences in blood sugar excursions. In 1932, Jean La Barre coined the term 'incretin' to refer to a then unknown hormone and hypothesised its release from the gut following a meal to enhance the release of insulin. The effects of the hypothesised incretin hormone on stabilising blood sugar became known as the 'incretin effect' (*fig 10.1*). The identity of the incretin hormones remained unknown for many decades to come. Then in the 1960s, a new radioimmunoassay for insulin revealed for the first time that insulin response to a sugar load (the rise in blood insulin levels following a meal) is two to three times greater when the same amount of sugar is ingested orally than when it is injected into a vein. This is what accounts for the relative stability of blood sugar when sugar is ingested orally compared to the same amount of sugar infused into a vein. Put simply, a bigger insulin response following orally ingested sugar means a smaller rise in blood sugar.

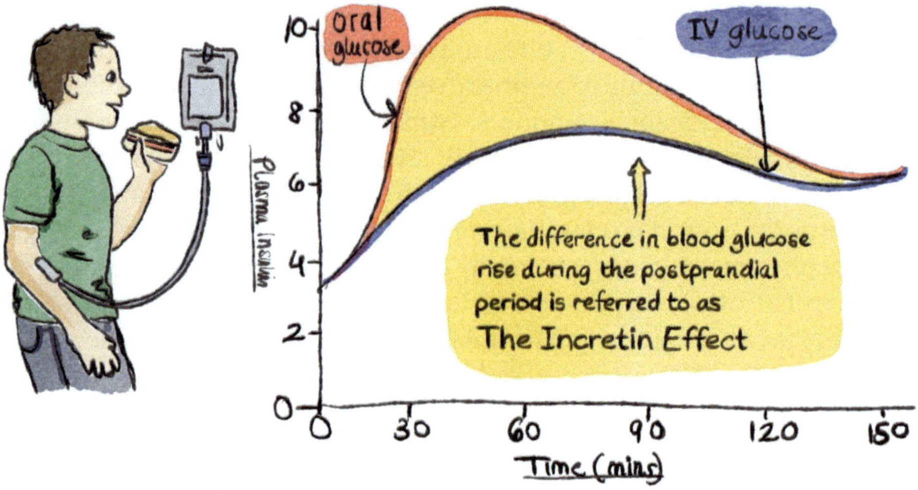

Figure 10.1: The 'Incretin Effect' (schematic [plasma insulin units for illustration only and are not accurate] based on data from Nauck et al. (2)). The incretin effect refers to the more pronounced insulin release in the postprandial period for oral glucose compared with intravenous glucose due to the effect of incretin hormones on insulin release with the former. The net result is a smaller postprandial blood glucose spike after oral ingestion of glucose compared with that following intravenous administration of glucose.

So far so good. We are up to the 1960s now, and we know about the 'incretin effect' as described and how this is mediated through differences in blood insulin responses following a sugar load, depending on its mode of administration. The theory at the time (as first hypothesised by Jean La Barre over 30 years earlier) was that there was some 'incretin factor' released from the gut in response to a sugar stimulus within the gut that is bypassed when sugar is administered into a vein (when the sugar load bypasses the gut). The nature of this 'incretin factor' though remained unknown. In the 1970s, the first 'incretin factor' was discovered and called 'Gastric Inhibitory Polypeptide' (GIP). Then, in the 1980s, the Gila monster waddles onto the scene, lifting its body high on its short legs and swinging its tail from side to side. But watch out for its bite! The Gila monster is the largest and only venomous lizard native to the United States and lives in the desert. In humans, the bite of the Gila monster can cause extreme pain, and it was this that attracted scientists to study its saliva, in which a molecule called 'exendin-4' was discovered. This discovery played a crucial role in the identification of the second major incretin hormone, GLP-1. Over the subsequent years and decades, there has been (and continues to be) intense research interest into the physiology and therapeutic potential of these two major incretin hormones, GIP and GLP-1. For the remainder of this chapter though, we will focus our attention on GLP-1, as this is the main peptide component of the 'skinny jabs' (and tablets) that are currently available and in development.

The Physiology of GLP-1

So much for the historical context. What about the physiology of GLP-1? To answer this question, we need to take a step back and look at the bigger picture. In Chapter 5, I discussed the interconnectedness between the gut (mediated by the gut microbiota) and the brain. The gut is one of the most complex endocrine systems in the body and one of the most highly innervated. ('Endocrine' refers to hormones that are chemical messengers that are released from a tissue and control cellular action, often in other tissues; 'Innervated' simply refers to the extent to which nerve endings supply a particular tissue.) What this means is that the gut is supremely well placed to communicate with the brain and peripheral organs like the liver, for example. Even with our modern-day insights though, our understanding of the gut is still in its infancy.

Our physiology is geared towards different modes of living. Regarding our gut physiology, the timing of the last meal is particularly relevant. When it comes to GLP-1, much of the action occurs during what is known as the 'postprandial period' that is the 3–4 hours that follow a meal. When you think about it, a lot of things need to happen simultaneously when we eat a meal, so the body can prepare itself for an onslaught of nutrients. A useful analogy here is to imagine a popular restaurant when it first opens for the evening. It will go from being empty to being full of customers in a relatively short time. During this transition phase, lots of things need to happen at the same time. The greeter needs to coordinate how many customers come into the restaurant to avoid overcrowding; the front-of-house staff needs to welcome the guests that are admitted, show them to their tables, provide the menu, take their orders, etc.; kitchen staff need to prepare the food for each order. This weird analogy likens the restaurant itself to the gut (primarily the stomach), the customers admitted likened to the food ingested, the head chef to the pancreatic β-cells that release insulin, the food served from the kitchen to the insulin released from the pancreas, the greeter on the front desk to our appetite, which influences how many customers are 'ingested' into the restaurant and our maitre d (Head Waiter, and the one in charge) to the main incretin hormone, GLP-1, coordinating the whole show. Our weird analogy plays out whilst the real effects of GLP-1 manifest within the postprandial phase of each customer during and after their meal! (Please bear with me on this one. I know it is not a perfect analogy and that in reality insulin does not interact with food in the stomach but rather acts later once the nutrients are absorbed into the blood, but this analogy will suffice for our purposes.) Following a meal and as soon as nutrients start to reach the small intestine (ileum), specialised cells release GLP-1 into the blood in response. In our analogy, this is like the customers entering the restaurant for the first time, and this is the moment when our maitre d awakens from his slumber and springs into action (I am assigning a 'he' for maitre d, but 'he' could just as easily be a 'she'). It is just as well our maitre d had a good sleep, as he has lots of work to do and lots of points of call, all happening simultaneously! Remember, the maitre d is the GLP-1 molecule in our analogy.

Although the postprandial effects of GLP-1 occur simultaneously, for ease I will describe them sequentially. GLP-1 stimulates insulin release from β-cells within the pancreas directly, and this results in a boost to the release of insulin. In our analogy, our maitre d barges into the kitchen, and he wakes up the head chef, shouting 'Cummon! Get a move on! We have got loads of customers arriving for their food. Work faster!' Importantly for our analogy though, our head chef is intelligent and has a window looking out into the restaurant and can see how many customers are waiting. He only responds to the maitre d if he can see that customers are waiting for food. In the same way, GLP-1 only elicits an insulin response from the β-cells if blood sugar is above a certain level. This has important implications for the therapeutic utility of the GLP-1 class, which generally avoid hypoglycaemia (low blood sugar levels). In the same way that GLP-1 stimulates insulin release from the β-cells, it also suppresses the release of a hormone called glucagon that is released from the pancreatic α-cells. (Let us think of glucagon as the deep cleaning staff in our analogy). Our maitre d tells all the deep cleaning staff with their mops and cleaning materials to go home until early the next day when the customers have left the restaurant, ready for the next deep clean.

Where to next for our poor little maitre d? Well, it is important to make sure that the customers are happy and have a good meal. Our maitre d doesn't want them walking out of the restaurant prematurely before they have been fed and so invests time in going around the seated customers to check they have their meals and drinks and that all is good. It is important for the maitre d to retain customers in the restaurant for the duration of their meal. In a similar way, GLP-1 slows down emptying of the stomach contents into the small intestine (duodenum), and this means that food stays in the stomach for longer after a meal, and this makes us feel full. At the same time though, our maitre d is acutely aware of potential customers queuing up on the street outside and so makes a beeline for the greeter on the door and tells them to slow down customer entry into the restaurant and possibly to send some people away. It is important for our maitre d to keep a check on how many customers are coming through the door, otherwise the restaurant could become overcrowded. This is the final main effect of GLP-1, to suppress our appetite directly within the hypothalamus and therefore ensure that we eventually stop eating to avoid over-filling our stomach. In our analogy, the greeter represents our appetite for food, and our maitre d acts like GLP-1 to suppress the greeter's 'appetite' to admit more customers into the restaurant (*fig 10.2*).

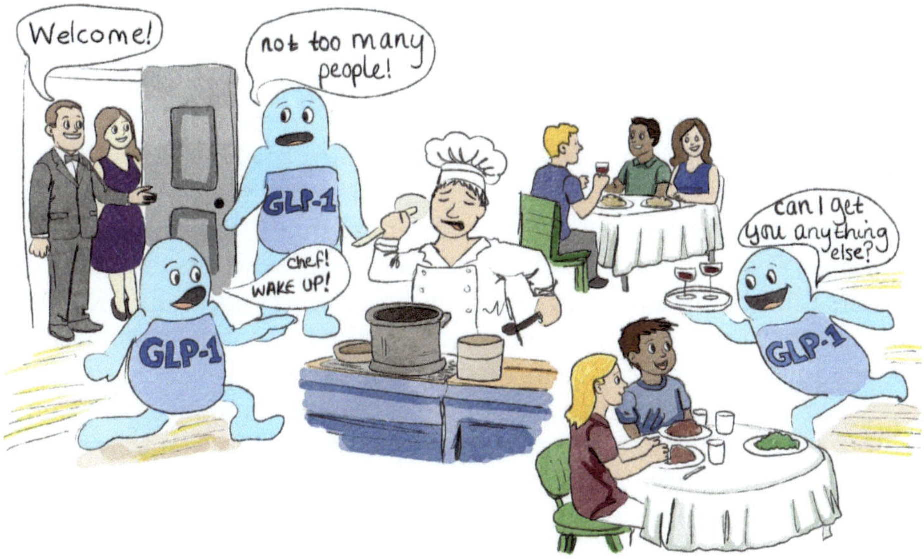

Figure 10.2: GLP-1 as the maitre d.

So, there you have it. GLP-1 physiology described here in just three paragraphs. To be clear, the receptors for GLP-1 are expressed in numerous tissues all over the body, and there are doubtless other GLP-1-related effects that are less well understood and that will emerge in the future. For our purposes though, what I describe here is what we need to know. If you want to understand GLP-1 physiology, just think of our maitre d, waking and chivvying the head chef, dismissing the deep cleaners, tending to (and retaining) the customers in the restaurant and keeping a close check on the greeter's 'appetite' to admit more customers into the restaurant. The net effect of this postprandial GLP-1 action is that the body is fully prepared for its ingested nutrients, with blood sugar levels that remain relatively constant (due to appropriate changes in insulin and glucagon release and delayed release of nutrients from the stomach into the duodenum), and an effective braking mechanism on our appetite and eating behaviour to stop us from eating too much food. Although beyond the scope of this chapter, insulin also plays a major role as the main anabolic hormone controlling assimilation of absorbed nutrients within the liver and their subsequent uptake and handling within peripheral tissues like fat and skeletal muscle, during the postprandial period.

Therapeutic Rationale and the Early Days of GLP-1-Based Therapies

Following these key insights into GLP-1 physiology, the next part of our story in the late 20th century involves researchers exploring how GLP-1 functions in people with T2D. Through comparing the incretin response to orally ingested sugar between those with T2D and controls, it was shown that in T2D there is 'incretin dysfunction'. To explain what this means, we need to go back to our restaurant analogy. Imagine this time that our maitre d is lazy. When the customers start coming in, he just can't be bothered to go into the kitchen to chivvy up the head chef. He doesn't really care whether the customers are well served, and the customers, as a result, leave the restaurant prematurely and dissatisfied. He doesn't bother to keep a check on the greeter who lets too many customers into the restaurant. The whole situation is a mess, and Kojak (in my opinion, the coolest TV detective) is called to come and investigate what's going on. Kojak appears on the scene and says in his characteristic American accent, 'Hey listen up. There's nothing wrong with these guys', pointing at the head chef, customers and greeter. He then points at the maitre d and shouts 'As for you, you are a lazy piece of excrement!', and with that he puts his lolly back in his mouth, puts on his trilby and casually walks out. As he walks past the restaurant manager on his way out, he quips 'just replace the lazy maitre d and everything will be fine'. The next day, the maitre d is replaced with one full of vim, energy and initiative, and Kojak's prediction comes true!

This story illustrates the original therapeutic rationale for GLP-1-based therapies. (I am confident that by now you have a good grounding in GLP-1 physiology and so will use this medically correct term instead of 'skinny jab'.) Essentially in T2D, GLP-1 does not work as well: analogous to our lazy maitre d. This is partly due to inadequate GLP-1 release in the postprandial period, and partly due to reduced effectiveness of GLP-1 at its receptor. This means that appetite is less well suppressed, food goes through the stomach quicker and less insulin is released after a meal. The net effect? Increases in blood glucose levels after a meal and increased food intake: Hallmarks of T2D. This provided the original rationale for development of GLP-1-based therapies for the glycaemic (sugar) management of T2D. The idea was to replace the deficient GLP-1 response in T2D with an exogenous injection (under the skin) of therapeutic GLP-1. In 2005, Exenatide was the first GLP-1-based therapy to be 'Food and Drug Administration' (FDA) approved for the glycaemic management of T2D. Exenatide is based on 'exendin-4', the molecule from the saliva of our old friend, the Gila monster. In 2007, Exenatide was first approved in the United Kingdom for use in T2D.

Since the launch of Exenatide, numerous other GLP-1 therapies were then launched, all for the licensed indication of improving glycaemic control in T2D. GLP-1s became a heterogeneous and unwieldy drug class, with some molecules (like Liraglutide) based on human GLP-1, others (like Exenatide) based on reptilian 'exendin-4', some being administered once a week, whilst others were administered more frequently. Other heterogeneity included efficacy regarding both glycaemic and weight-loss effects and improvement in cardiovascular outcomes. Most GLP-1 therapies launched were injectable, with one (Rybelsus) being an oral form of (injectable) Semaglutide.

The Modern Era of GLP-1-Based Therapies

In 2017, there was a shift in emphasis for the therapeutic indication of the GLP-1-based therapies. Instead of purely focusing on their glycaemic effects in T2D, some of these therapies had a change in licensing for weight loss in the context of obesity (outside of T2D). To go back to our restaurant analogy, 2017 marked a time when our attention shifted away from the effects of the maitre d on the head chef (insulin release) to his effects on the greeter (appetite control). The first GLP-1-based drug to be licensed for weight loss in obesity was Saxenda. At this point, I need to provide some clarity on nomenclature. Saxenda is Liraglutide in high-dose form. The same molecule, Liraglutide, in its lower-dose form is called Victoza. The company, Novo Nordisk chose to use different names, Saxenda and Victoza, for the same molecule (but different doses) to discern between their different licensing, for obesity and T2D, respectively.

Next on the scene in the United Kingdom in 2019 was Semaglutide, a weekly form of GLP-1. As with Liraglutide, Semaglutide was launched initially as Ozempic and licensed for use in T2D, and then in 2023 was launched in high-dose form as Wegovy for its weight-loss effects in obesity. Also, in the same year, we had the launch of Tirzepatide (Mounjaro) as the first 'dual-incretin agonist', with effects on both GLP-1 and GIP. To date, Tirzepatide has been licensed primarily for T2D, although there are plans issued by the National Institute for Health and Care Excellence (NICE) in the United Kingdom for it to become available to 3.5M people living with obesity in the UK population over the next 12-years. However, the details of this plan have yet to be confirmed at the time of writing.

Globally, 'Big Pharma' dominates the GLP-1-based drug market currently and is likely to in years to come with impressive portfolios of novel drugs in various phases of development and yet to be launched. As indicated earlier, many biotechnology companies have an interest in therapies that induce weight loss, including through GLP-1-based effects. Over the coming years, we will see numerous new classes of GLP-1-based therapies and other classes of weight-loss therapies being launched, and the obesity field will become quite crowded. At the time of writing, the two main GLP-1-based therapies being used for weight-loss purposes in obesity are Wegovy (Semaglutide) and Mounjaro (Tirzepatide, also

Table 10.1: Currently available GLP-1 therapies licensed for obesity

Molecule	Trade name	Molecule type	Injection frequency	Dosing	Body weight loss potential
Liraglutide	Saxenda	GLP-1 agonist	Daily	0.6 mg–3 mg	Up to 10%
Semaglutide	Wegovy	GLP-1 agonist	Weekly	0.25 mg–2.4 mg	Up to 15%
Tirzepatide	Mounjaro	GLP-1-GIP dual agonist	Weekly	2.5 mg–15 mg	Up to 22.5%

GIP: Gastric Inhibitory Polypeptide; GLP-1: Glucagon-Like Peptide-1

known as Zepbound in the United States). Each of these is administered (usually self-administered) through a weekly injection given under the skin. (Wegovy is also available as a tablet). Each has its own titration regimen, which usually involves starting at a low dose and gradually increasing each month to a maximum tolerated dose. In the case of Mounjaro, the titration phase can last up to 5-months. Although these two therapies are different in their molecular design, there are commonalities between these and other GLP-1 therapies (*Table 10.1*).

I have extensive clinical experience and expertise in prescribing GLP-1 therapies to thousands of my patients since this drug class was launched nearly 20-years ago. In the next section, I will use my own personal insights and data from the current medical literature to answer some commonly asked questions about Wegovy and Mounjaro.

What Are the Safety Concerns with GLP-1 Therapies?

Before starting a drug like Wegovy or Mounjaro, there are potential safety concerns that need to be properly addressed by your healthcare professional. I can't stress enough that these therapies are not commodities. They are serious and highly specialised drug therapies, which should only be taken if prescribed by a suitably qualified healthcare professional, and if appropriate medical assessment and follow-up is in place. This would usually be a specialist endocrinologist or your GP (family doctor). Certain preclusions include a history of pancreatitis or risk factors for pancreatitis (such as alcohol excess, gallstones, or raised triglycerides [a type of fat in the blood]). Also, any history of medullary thyroid cancer in either you or your family members would preclude use of a GLP-1 therapy. Pregnancy and breastfeeding are contraindications, and for women of childbearing age, reliable contraception should be used. For Mounjaro, recent guidance advises that the efficacy of the oral contraceptive pill can be diminished, and so use of barrier forms of contraception is therefore recommended. For patients with T2D, some forms of retinopathy can also be a contraindication to the use of GLP-1 therapies. If pancreatitis occurs whilst on a GLP-1 therapy, the therapy would normally be discontinued immediately and no further GLP-1 therapies used as a precaution. It should be noted, however, that the number of people who develop pancreatitis on GLP-1 therapies is extremely low, and this potential rare side effect is not proven beyond doubt. If you are on a GLP-1 therapy and you become unwell with upper abdominal and/or back pain and/or persistent vomiting, then you need to seek immediate medical attention, as pancreatitis is a serious condition (sometimes even fatal) requiring immediate hospital-based medical management.

What Are the Tolerability Concerns of GLP-1 Therapies?

The main tolerability concerns for Wegovy and Mounjaro are upper gastrointestinal (GI) side effects of nausea (feeling sick) and vomiting and occasionally diarrhoea and constipation. You will likely feel full for longer (due to delayed gastric [stomach] emptying), and this may result in eructation (burping). Your taste sensation may become diminished somewhat and you may enjoy food less. These upper GI side effects are usually mild or moderate in intensity and generally wear off after around 8–12-weeks of being on the GLP-1 therapy. If these symptoms become too troublesome, there may be the option of reducing the dose (as these effects are usually dose-dependent), and this may improve tolerability. Occasionally, you may need to stop a GLP-1 therapy if GI intolerance is severe enough, but that would be unusual.

How Much Weight Loss Will I Achieve with a GLP-1 Therapy?

Recently, a trial was published that answers this very question. It can be difficult to make comparisons for different drugs across multiple trials. However, 'SURMOUNT-5' was a direct head-to-head trial to assess the weight-loss effects of Wegovy versus Mounjaro in participants with obesity (without T2D) over 72-weeks. It was shown that the average weight loss for Wegovy was around 14% and for Mounjaro was around 20% (3). It is important to state though that these are average weight loss responses across participants within the trial. We know from this and other trials that whenever a GLP-1 is used, there is usually a spectrum of weight loss responses, with around 10% of participants being 'super-responders', around 10% being 'non-responders' and the remaining 80% having a weight loss response somewhere between these two extremes. Unfortunately, we are unable currently to determine who will respond in what way prior to initiating the therapy (although in future we may be able to gain some insight from genetic analysis of the GLP-1 receptor). We do know, however, that if you have T2D, then your weight loss response to a GLP-1 therapy will likely be less pronounced than that for people who do not have T2D. Furthermore, if you are a woman, you will likely, on average, lose more weight with a GLP-1 therapy compared with the weight loss response to GLP-1 therapy in men. The other important point here, as I discussed in Chapter 4, is that through the induction of a 'negative energy balance' with a GLP-1 therapy (from reduced caloric intake), although most body weight loss stems from fat tissue, between 15% and 25% of body weight loss is from the lean tissues (primarily the skeletal muscles). Reduced skeletal muscle mass can worsen overall metabolic health and is a problem with all GLP-1-based therapies, but particularly those with the greatest amount of weight loss potential like Wegovy and Mounjaro. There are lifestyle strategies that can mitigate against this problem, and novel skeletal muscle-focused therapies in development, as I discussed in detail in Chapter 4.

How Long Can I Take a GLP-1 Therapy for?

This is an open question and depends on multiple factors. Some of my patients who are on GLP-1 therapies have been on them for many years. From a medical perspective, there is no time limit on these therapies and no logical reason why they can only be prescribed for a pre-defined time period. Provided that the therapy remains efficacious and is well tolerated and there are no safety concerns, then it is usually fine to continue to take the therapy. It is important that when taking a GLP-1 therapy, there is regular and ongoing medical review from a qualified healthcare professional, who can then advise on the plan going forward, possible change of dose and whether to continue or stop the therapy. There are certain scenarios in which the therapy should be discontinued immediately, for example if pancreatitis develops or if pregnancy occurs. Previously, NICE provided time limits on the use of some GLP-1 therapies in obesity (but not when used for T2D), including 2- years. Such guidelines are likely driven by health-economic reasons. There is no logical medical reason why GLP-1 therapies should be discontinued after only 2-years when used for obesity! Finally, if you are self-funding a GLP-1 therapy, then the ongoing costs of the therapy may place a limit on how long you can continue it due to affordability.

What Happens to My Weight When I Stop a GLP-1 Therapy?

I am afraid that I am not going to be the bearer of good news with this one. Unfortunately, the reported studies (and my own professional anecdotal experience) of what happens after stopping a GLP-1 therapy consistently show a regain in body weight. It gets worse though. As I discussed in Chapter 4, you will likely regain more fat than skeletal muscle, and so your overall body composition may get a bit worse. The amount of weight regain is variable, and you may not regain all the weight that you lost whilst on the GLP-1, but it is likely that you will regain at least some of it. This process happens usually over a few weeks and months. The reason is that whilst you were on the GLP-1, your appetite was being suppressed, and then when you come off it, there is a sudden release of the brake on your appetite, and you feel hungry again. As I discussed in Chapter 2, your appetite will likely have become enhanced with weight loss, and so there is a double whammy blow to your appetite control (or lack of it). Going back to our restaurant analogy, whilst taking the GLP-1, you have a turbo-charged maitre d who is overly officious with the greeter, preventing admission of new customers into the restaurant with the result that loads of potential customers start queuing up outside. That's the suppressed appetite kicking in. Once you stop the GLP-1 therapy, the maitre d suddenly becomes sleepy, and the greeter starts letting all the queuing customers into the restaurant. This is the reactivation of your previously suppressed appetite (which becomes enhanced on stopping GLP-1 therapy due to the prior GLP-1-induced weight loss). Weight regain on stopping a GLP-1 therapy is not inevitable and depends on a few factors, including how much weight you lost whilst taking the GLP-1. If you can maintain your healthy diet, eating behaviour and lifestyle, then this will help, although I appreciate that this is easier said than done if your enhanced appetite drives you to eat more food! The reality is that most of us cannot consciously override an enhanced appetite. In fact, the misconception that we can consciously override our appetite seems widespread and likely contributes towards societal negative attitudes towards those who live with obesity and its stigmatisation.

How Does a GLP-1 Therapy Help Me to Lose Weight?

GLP-1 therapies have multiple effects. However, to answer this question we just need to know about two of them. The first is that GLP-1 therapies act directly in the hypothalamus (an area of the brain) to suppress appetite. This means that our drive to eat food is diminished, and we are less interested in food, and so we eat less. It is like the maitre d keeping a very close check on the greeter who in turn lets in only a trickle of customers through the restaurant door. The other main GLP-1 effect occurs within the stomach, to slow emptying of nutrients into the small intestine. This is like the maitre d ensuring that the customers stay in the restaurant for longer, to enable a more relaxed meal. This has the effect of making you feel fuller earlier during a meal and helps you to avoid overeating. There are data to suggest that GLP-1 can act on the taste receptors in the tongue to diminish their receptivity, meaning that food doesn't taste as good, and this can also contribute towards a reduced appetite.

Beyond Weight Loss, Are There Other Health Benefits of Taking a GLP-1 Therapy?

Yes! Obesity contributes towards >50 weight-related conditions. Effective weight loss will likely improve the outcomes of all of these. Remember that GLP-1 therapies were designed and launched initially for the treatment of T2D and specifically to improve glycaemic (sugar) control. There are also improvements in blood pressure and blood cholesterol levels. In addition to these benefits, we should also give a mention to improvement in overall risk of having a cardiovascular event (like a heart attack or stroke). In the SELECT trial, it was shown that the use of Wegovy in obesity for those who have already had a cardiovascular event significantly reduces the risk of having another cardiovascular event (4). At the time of writing, the cardiovascular outcome trials for Mounjaro in obesity have not yet been published, and these trials are in progress.

The Future of Obesity Management

I am going to conclude this chapter with a brief overview of the future of pharmacotherapies for obesity. The Roman god Janus is quite apt for our purposes here. Janus had two faces, one looking back and one looking forward, and was used to denote a portal or gateway. Looking back at the obesity pharmacotherapy field prior to 2017, Janus sees the history of pharmacotherapies for obesity as impoverished and chequered, with examples of therapies launched and then subsequently withdrawn for various reasons, and those that were available typically had a weight loss of between 3% and 5%. Looking forward though, Janus sees the obesity pharmacotherapy field with an exciting and propitious future. Now the benchmark for weight loss with pharmacotherapies has been raised above 20%, and who knows how high it will become.

Traditionally, weight loss management consists of three elements: lifestyle (including dietary) modification, pharmacotherapy and bariatric surgery. Although lifestyle should be applied throughout, bariatric surgery has always been considered as 'end of the line', to be used if all else fails. Furthermore, the weight loss potential of bariatric surgery has always far exceeded that of pharmacotherapies. However, we have now entered an era in which the latest iterations of GLP-1-based therapies are almost on a par with some forms of bariatric surgery (such as sleeve gastrectomy) regarding their weight loss potential. This will likely require us to modify our future algorithms of obesity management and consider some pharmacotherapies more on an equal footing with some forms of bariatric surgery regarding their weight loss potential. This will have implications for the way in which obesity management is structured and administered.

At the time of writing, we have three available GLP-1 therapies that are used for obesity management in the United Kingdom: Saxenda, Wegovy and Mounjaro. Over the coming years and decades, we will see the launch of multiple novel GLP-1-based therapies. These therapies are being designed in a way to combine therapeutic effects of multiple intestinal hormones (5). What happens typically is that a single molecule is designed with sequences attached that mimic separate incretin and intestinal hormones. In this way, a single molecule can have effects on multiple different receptors simultaneously. Mounjaro is one example of a single molecule that elicits effects at both GLP-1 and GIP receptors. Another example is Retatrutide (at the time of writing, still in development and yet to be launched), which is a 'triple incretin agonist' and consists of a single molecule with sequences that represent GLP-1, GIP and glucagon hormones. (Hang on a second, I hear you say! Isn't glucagon released from the α-cells in the pancreas and suppressed by GLP-1? That is correct, but another intestinal hormone called Oxyntomodulin, released following a meal, has glucagon-like effects through acting on the glucagon receptor.) It turns out that stimulation of glucagon receptors within the liver postprandially enhance lipid oxidation and reduce liver fat. Retatrutide has not only excellent weight loss effects but also remarkable effects at reducing liver fat. There are other dual incretin agonists that combine GLP-1 with glucagon (such as Survodutide) that are also effective at improving both body weight and liver fat.

Fatty liver, or 'Metabolic Dysfunction-Associated Fatty Liver Disease' (MAFLD) to give it its proper medical name, is an extremely important metabolic sequela of obesity. MAFLD is incredibly common, with some estimates suggesting a prevalence of up to 1 in 3 of the world's adult population. It is beyond the scope of this chapter to discuss this topic in depth. Suffice it to say that MAFLD has now overtaken alcohol excess as the world's leading cause of cirrhosis. Although it typically takes decades for cirrhosis to develop from MAFLD, and perhaps <1%

of those with MAFLD ultimately end up with cirrhosis, the global prevalence of MAFLD is such that unless we act now, we will sleepwalk into a tsunami of MAFLD-related cirrhosis and other forms of serious liver-related disease in decades to come. The good news is that the liver has a remarkable regenerative capacity, and if we can use therapies to reduce substantially the amount of fat in the liver, then we can potentially have a major impact on the global burden of cirrhosis in the future. This is one reason why novel therapies like Retatrutide and other molecules that incorporate glucagon (like Survodutide) have such great potential for the future management of obesity. In our future approach to the management of obesity, we need to look beyond weight loss per se, to the effective management of the metabolic sequelae of obesity, including MAFLD.

There is a lot of interest regarding the 'glipron' class, which are molecules that are designed to have similar actions to GLP-1, but which can be taken by mouth and at any time of day regardless of meals. This is because the glipron molecules are 'non-peptidic', meaning that they are not peptides and therefore do not consist of a string of amino acids (as is the case for native GLP-1, and other incretin and intestinal hormones). Glipron molecules are therefore resistant to enzymes like peptidases in the stomach that would otherwise break them down before being absorbed. These therapies show great potential and could help to transition towards a more community-based focus for obesity management, given their ease of prescription (without the need for a nurse to show the patient how to use the injection device, for example). The first of the giiprons to be launched is Orforglipron (recently FDA-approved in the United States as Foundayo at the time of writing). There is also a lot of interest in the effects of amylin, which is co-released with insulin from the pancreatic β-cells, and has similar effects to GLP-1 including appetite suppression but via different receptors. There is a drug called Cagrisema that combines cagrilintide (a long-acting amylin analogue) with Semaglutide, which has great weight loss potential, and other amylin analogues at various stages of development. Finally, there is a molecule called MariTide that combines an agonist of GLP-1 (stimulates the GLP-1 receptor), and wait for it, an antagonist of GIP (suppresses action at the GIP receptor). I know this is confusing given how Mounjaro works, but the evidence for this molecule shows good weight loss effects that seem to last for weeks or even months after just one dose. We are still trying to figure out the mechanism, but if these long-lasting effects play out in subsequent trials, this molecule could perhaps play a useful role in mitigating against weight regain following discontinuation of GLP-1 therapies in the future (*fig 10.3*).

To finish, I am going to go right back to the start. Believe it or not, the first ever weight loss drug was used way back in the 1930s. This drug

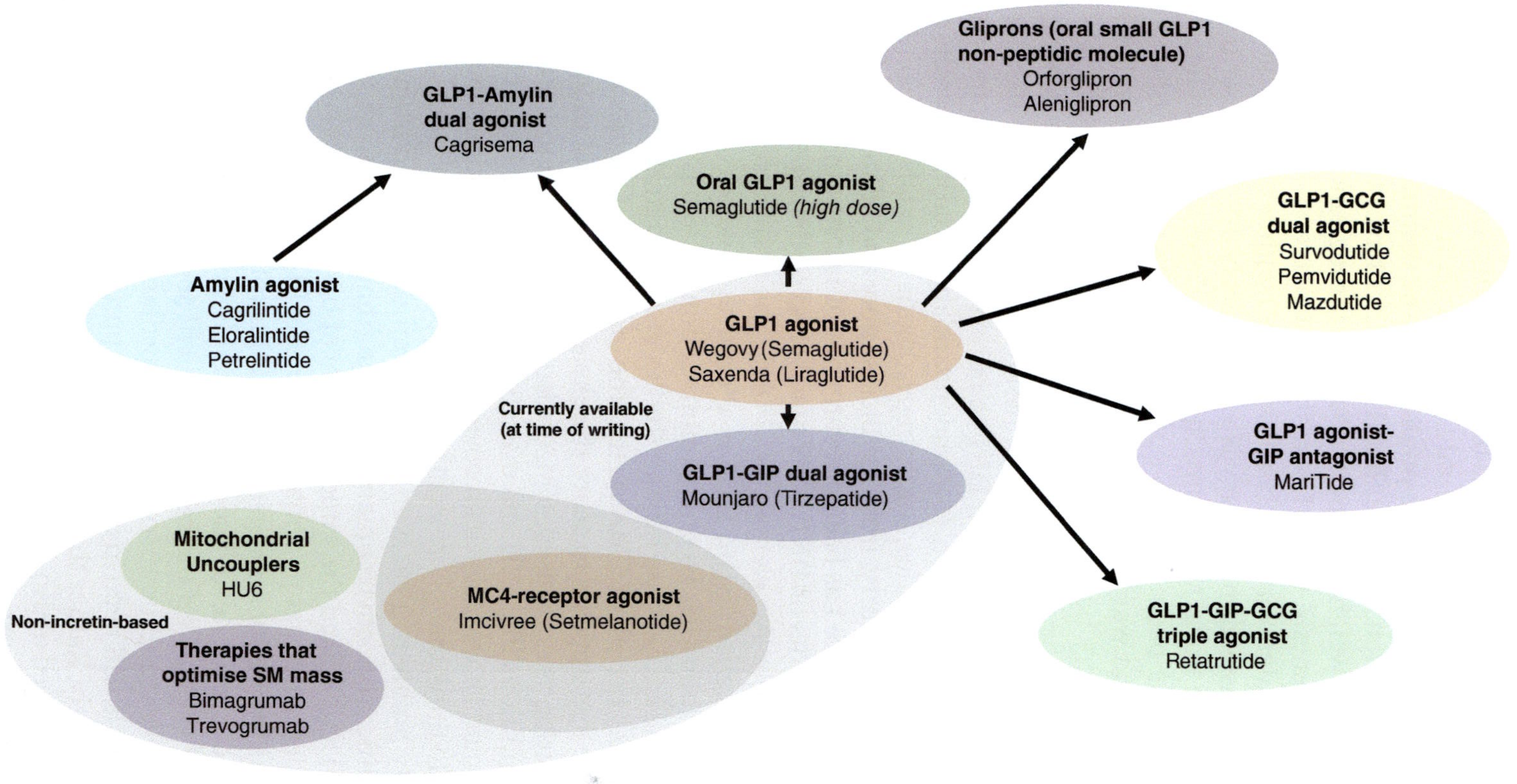

Figure 10.3: The future of obesity management. GCG, Glucagon; GIP, Gastric Inhibitory Polypeptide; GLP1, Glucagon-Like Peptide-1; MC4, Melanocortin 4; SM, Skeletal Muscle. (Technically, amylin is not an incretin hormone as it does not stimulate insulin release, but it has many other properties of incretin hormones, including suppression of appetite). Imcivree (Setmelanotide) is only currently licensed and indicated for certain rare genetic and syndromic forms of obesity. Oral semaglutide (Rybelsus) is currently licensed for Type 2 Diabetes Mellitus, but not for obesity.

has nothing to do with GLP-1. It is called '2,4-Dinitrophenol' (DNP) and has an explosive history, having been used in munitions in World War 1. Incredibly, back in the 1930s (around the time that the term 'incretin' was coined), DNP was sold to the public 'over the counter' and didn't even need a prescription. Imagine that! How times have changed. DNP undoubtedly causes weight loss (6). It does this through inducing a process called thermogenesis, which I described in Chapter 4. DNP inhibits the production of Adenosine Triphosphate (ATP) within the mitochondria of cells, and instead this energy is released as heat (remember the rogue worker in the Royal Mint from Chapter 4). There is even an anecdote of DNP having been used by Russian soldiers to prevent hypothermia during World War 2 (6). The problem (and it is a huge problem) is that DNP has a very narrow 'therapeutic index', meaning that it is easy to die from it if the dose is not exactly right, and there are reports of fatalities. DNP therefore was withdrawn from the market in 1938, at which time the US FDA declared DNP to be 'extremely dangerous and not fit for human consumption' (6). Understandably, pharma interest in DNP waned for many decades. Alarmingly, deaths from DNP appear to have resurfaced this century, from its illicit supply and administration.

In recent times, there has been a resurgence of interest in the potential therapeutic benefits of DNP. This novel class of therapies is called 'Controlled Metabolic Accelerators' (CMAs). The first in class CMA is a small molecule called 'HU6'. HU6 is a 'prodrug' and is converted to DNP in the liver following its oral administration. HU6 has undergone rodent-based and early-phase human studies to assess its safety and tolerability. One key benefit of CMAs is that the induced weight loss comes from fat tissue and appears to spare the skeletal muscle, and therefore body composition is optimised. CMAs also have potential to improve metabolic conditions like T2D and overall cardiometabolic health (7).

In this chapter, I have focused on obesity pharmacotherapies. It would be a mistake to think that pharmacotherapies provide the solution to the global obesity problem. That would be to diminish the importance of lifestyle modification, environmental change (that I will discuss in the final chapter) and indeed the important role of bariatric surgery. However, it is undeniable that pharmacotherapies will continue to play an important role in obesity management, and this role will likely grow in the years and decades ahead. There are many challenges. With multiple new classes of therapy on the horizon, we will soon have a multitude of novel therapies (and new drug classes) available to us, and healthcare professionals will need to choose these appropriately and combine them imaginatively. Rather than one-size-fits-all, we will need to adopt a more individualised approach to obesity management, with a bespoke selection of therapies according to the specific and unique needs of individuals (doubtless with the support of algorithms powered by artificial intelligence). These needs are many and varied, discussed throughout this and other chapters, including cardiovascular risk, degree of MAFLD, presence of T2D, state of skeletal muscle, ability to engage in resistance physical exercise and heart function. Whichever approach we take, we need to optimise body composition and move away from our current obsession with overall body weight loss and Body Mass Index. Our future therapeutic armamentarium should enable us to achieve this important aim. The incretin pathway may no longer be a new therapeutic target for obesity. But it is certainly one that is here to stay.

References

1. Barber TM, Begbie H, Levy J. The incretin pathway as a new therapeutic target for obesity. Maturitas. 2010;67(3):197–202.
2. Nauck M, Stöckmann F, Ebert R, Creutzfeldt W. Reduced incretin effect in type 2 (non-insulin-dependent) diabetes. Diabetologia. 1986;29:46–52.
3. Aronne LJ, Horn DB, le Roux CW, Ho W, Falcon BL, Gomez Valderas E, et al. Tirzepatide as compared with semaglutide for the treatment of obesity. N Engl J Med. 2025;393(1):26–36.
4. Lincoff AM, Brown-Frandsen K, Colhoun HM, Deanfield J, Emerson SS, Esbjerg S, et al. Semaglutide and cardiovascular outcomes in obesity without diabetes. N Engl J Med. 2023;389(24):2221–32.
5. Statham L, Pelling M, Hanson P, Kyrou I, Randeva H, Barber TM. Designer GLP1 poly-agonist peptides in the management of diabesity. Expert Rev Endocrinol Metab. 2023;18(3):231–40.
6. Grundlingh J, Dargan PI, El-Zanfaly M, Wood DM. 2,4-Dinitrophenol (DNP): a weight loss agent with significant acute toxicity and risk of death. J Med Toxicol. 2011;7(3):205–12.
7. Noureddin M, Khan S, Portell F, Jorkasky D, Dennis J, Khan O, et al. Safety and efficacy of once-daily HU6 versus placebo in people with non-alcoholic fatty liver disease and high BMI: a randomised, double-blind, placebo-controlled, phase 2a trial. Lancet Gastroenterol Hepatol. 2023;8(12):1094–105.

11 Which Diet? Why No Size Fits All

Food, glorious food!

When I went to primary school as a very young lad (another school anecdote, but the last one of the book), quite a long time ago now, I had school meals. Once you had finished what you could eat, you handed your plate to the 'dinner nanny' (that is what they were called back then), who then tipped and scraped all the leftovers into a big black cylindrical bin, the contents of which were sent for pig feed at the end of each day. I daresay the pigs were delighted with this arrangement. Thinking back to the sight and smell of the bin contents, particularly if you were on '4th sittings' when the bin got quite full, turns my stomach to this day. On one occasion, I could not finish the roast potatoes on my plate, as they were disgusting. When I took my plate for 'slop out' the dinner nanny on duty that day was not happy. She decided that rather than allowing the pigs the joy of eating the roasts left on my plate, I would have to eat them all up myself, which being around 8 years old at the time, I duly did. (I almost vomited them into the pig-swill bin on my way out of the canteen, incidentally.) It was one of the low points of my school career, and for years afterwards, I could not eat roast potatoes because of that experience. In the spirit of the Lord Chancellor from Iolanthe (Gilbert and Sullivan, 1882: OK, I am not that old!), 'And I'll never eat roasts for the rest of my life. Said I to myself - said I'. I am sure you will be delighted to learn that, nowadays, I love eating roast potatoes and have now got over that negative childhood experience.

When I see patients in my obesity clinic, it is relatively common for some of them to recount negative food experiences. Often, these are childhood experiences and can be harrowing to listen to and sometimes redolent of abuse. We use food in all kinds of unpleasant ways, including as punishment or as a form of control. We also use food as an expression of love and even to represent love. Our relationship with food is unique to each of us. This relationship develops in a myriad of complex ways and influences all aspects of our lives in ways that may not even be apparent to us. Our experiences in childhood can often affect us profoundly as adults, and this includes our food preferences, diet and eating-related behaviours. Beyond our past experiences, there are other factors that may influence our food preferences. People can experience 'hypersensitivity' to environmental stimuli. This can be a feature of conditions like autism and 'Attention Deficit Hyperactivity Disorder' (ADHD) and can affect our taste sensation, with an aversion to strong and powerful tastes and a preference for milder-tasting foods.

In this chapter, I tackle the thorny topic of diet. By 'diet' what I mean is the food that we eat, but I will broaden this definition to include our eating-related behaviours. I will also dissect the idea of 'going on a diet', which to most people means a special or 'fad' diet, designed for a purpose, most commonly perhaps to lose weight. I will discuss the distractors that can thwart our attempts to eat healthily and leave us discombobulated. I will argue that our dietary needs and preferences are unique to each of us, but that generic expert dietary advice can go a long way.

And with that preamble, it is time to open our dietary Pandora's box, and see what delights await....

Distraction and Discombobulation

Have you ever noticed that there are so many food and diet experts out there? You only need to browse around the popular bookshelves in shops or peruse social media streams or even mainstream media to see that when it comes to food and diet, everyone is an expert. We all have our own perceived wisdom regarding diets, which may have been handed down to us from parents and grandparents. We all grew up with familiar mantras relating to food, such as the importance of eating our breakfast every morning, and not going to bed on an empty stomach, and these are internalised as children and stay with us as adults as accepted fact, never to be questioned. The reality is that we know far less about our food and nutrition than we think we know, and the food and diet myths that we all grew up with often have little if any supportive scientific evidence and frequently turn out to be untrue. Furthermore, it is remarkable that the drugs that we take are regulated, scrutinised and monitored highly, and rightly so. And yet, when it comes to the food that we eat, the regulation, scrutinisation and monitoring simply does not compare to that of drug therapies. This is ironic when one considers that unhealthy diets are an important contributor to obesity and much modern-day chronic ill health globally, to such a degree that is a million miles away from the cumulative health implications of adverse effects from drugs.

It is not surprising that as a species, we are obsessed with food. We need to eat to survive. Eating is an essential part of living and is usually enjoyable and often a social activity. Ever since we learnt how to control fire and the art of cooking our food, we have been obsessed with recipes, how to maximise the tastiness of our food, its nutritional value and our enjoyment of eating it. Our obsession with food underlies the extensive coverage and airtime devoted to food-related television programmes, magazines and newspaper articles (not to mention social media outlets). Eating food is one of the great pleasures of life and should be a joyous experience. It is a good thing that we have so many food-related programmes, with the proviso of course that they promote healthy recipes. It is also a good thing that food features so prominently in our culture. However, in our modern-day 'Information Revolution' age, there are multiple factors that can distract and confuse us and detract us from eating a healthy diet. One of these is our obsession with the kcal.

The 'kcal' stands for kilocalorie. The kcal is colloquially known simply as the 'calorie', and we use both 'kcal' and 'calorie' interchangeably on food labels. This is confusing. For ease, I will refer to the 'kcal' as 'calorie' for the rest of this chapter. What is a calorie? It is simply a measure of the energy content of our food. Scientifically, 1 calorie (kcal) is the amount of energy needed to raise 1 kg (1 litre) of water by 1°C, but that information is not particularly helpful to us when we are trying to make sense of this ubiquitously expressed measure in everyday life (*fig 11.1*). (I do not think many of us have in mind a kg of water with a thermometer placed in it atop a tripod, gauze and Bunsen burner when we are doing our supermarket shopping!) When we talk about the energy content of our food, we are referring to a special form of energy called 'chemical energy'. This is the energy contained within the molecular bonds holding all the atoms together

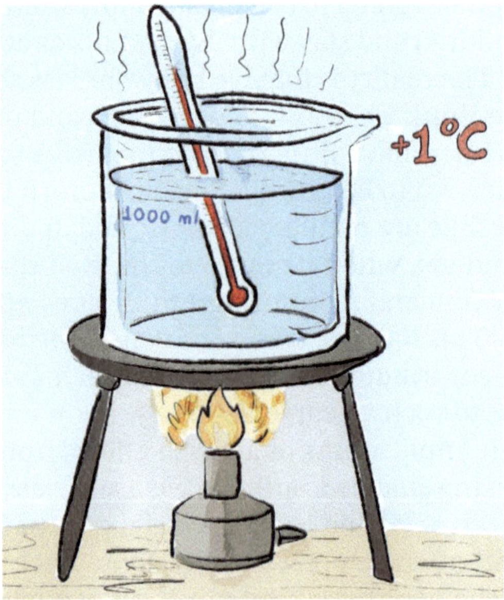

Figure 11.1: The calorie.

within our food. Following digestion and assimilation of our nutrients within the liver, the individual components of our food (broadly carbohydrates [sugar], fats and protein) reach our cells via the blood, and within our cells, their molecular bonds are broken down, and the energy released is used to power all the activities that go on in our cells all the time. This process underlies our metabolism. Importantly, all our food (even so-called 'calorie-negative' foods like celery) contains calories. Although fat leads the way with calories, containing 9 calories per gram, it may surprise you to learn that protein has the same caloric content as carbohydrate (sugar) at 4 calories per gram.

Our obsession with calories distracts and confuses us. Recently, I watched a documentary about a well-known chocolate maker based in the West Midlands in the United Kingdom, that had produced a bar of chocolate with 30% less sugar. Despite having less sugar, the caloric content of the chocolate had not changed appreciably. During the documentary, there was a question asked to someone (not from the company) to compare the taste of the reduced-sugar chocolate with the original chocolate. During the interview, she asked herself a question as to how it could be that the new chocolate bar had less sugar content and yet had a similar caloric content to the original chocolate bar and was genuinely confused by this. I mention this not to mock or to ridicule. Quite the opposite. I empathise with her and believe that her confusion is a good illustration of how our obsession with calories distracts and confuses us regarding our food. I dare say that a good proportion of the population would also be confused by this conundrum. The solution is that all food contains calories, not just sugar. By reducing sugar content in the chocolate, there is requisite replacement of that sugar with another ingredient: the reduced sugar cannot just exist as a vacuum within the chocolate; it needs replacement with some other sugar substitute. Although not sugar, this sugar substitute still contains calories, which is why there can be a reduction of sugar content whilst caloric content remains unchanged appreciably.

To be clear, I am not dismissing calories as a useless measure. Contrarily, caloric measures can be quite useful to gauge the energy content of our food. My point is that the calorie is just one measure of our food – one of multiple measures. And caloric content provides us with little insight into the nutritional value of our food. The problem is that we have become so obsessed by the calorie that we may judge our food solely by its caloric content, represented by a single number. Quite commonly now, when we buy food from an outlet, it will have the caloric content of that food item displayed prominently, as a 'guide' to whether we should choose it. The caloric content of our food is not a particularly useful way to judge the healthiness or nutritional quality of it. Remember that all food contains calories, even healthy food. If the caloric content of our food is our sole guide, then we could eat an unhealthy diet whilst ticking the calorie box and lull ourselves into a false sense of security. This is not helpful. Unfortunately, government 'targets' have contributed towards our caloric obsession. This includes 'guidance' that tells us the maximum number of calories we should eat each day, and these are sex-specific, with one figure for men and one figure for women. Not only does this approach promulgate our caloric obsession, this 'guidance' also suggests that the caloric requirements of every man are the same and ditto for every woman – a sex-specific 'one-size-fits-all' approach to our caloric needs. This is wrong. We are all individuals with daily caloric requirements that are unique to each of us (influenced by factors like our skeletal muscle (SM) mass, physical activity levels, age and multiple other dynamic factors).

Beyond our caloric obsession, we live in a culture in which there are a myriad of fad diets, each promoted by its own celebrity or influencer, and each with its fake promises of weight loss and other health benefits. There are fad diets that advocate cutting out all fat, others that advocate cutting out all carbohydrates, yet others that advocate eating raw liver or maximising protein intake, and innumerable other examples. These fad diets often have little if any scientific evidence backing up their various health claims. Then, to cap it all, we have some media streams publicising the latest data for a particular food item, with a sensationalist approach to reporting. With all these distractions, false claims and promises regarding fad diets, government 'guidance' on maximum daily caloric intake and sensationalised reporting on the latest epidemiological food-related studies, we are like rabbits startled in the headlights. We are bombarded by so much information, disinformation, misinformation and 'guidance' about our food and diet and calories on an almost daily basis that it is easy for us to become confused and respond with 'action-anxiety', in which we are anxious to eat anything in case it harms us or exceeds our 'one-sex-size-fits-all' daily caloric maximum allowance. This situation is redolent of the COVID-19 pandemic, in which the laws on what we could and could not do in the United Kingdom seemed to change almost every day, and everyone became confused and anxious about doing anything or going anywhere in case they broke the law. 'Do this, do not do that, do not go there....' When it comes to our food, 'action-anxiety' is not a good thing, as it may prevent us from eating a healthy and diverse diet. 'Action-anxiety' reminds me of a quote from a previous American president, Theodore Roosevelt, who said: 'In any moment of decision, the best thing you can do is the right thing, the next best thing is the wrong thing, and the worst thing you can do is nothing'. 'Action-anxiety' tends to place us in this final category and leaves us prone to doing nothing about our diet (*fig 11.2*).

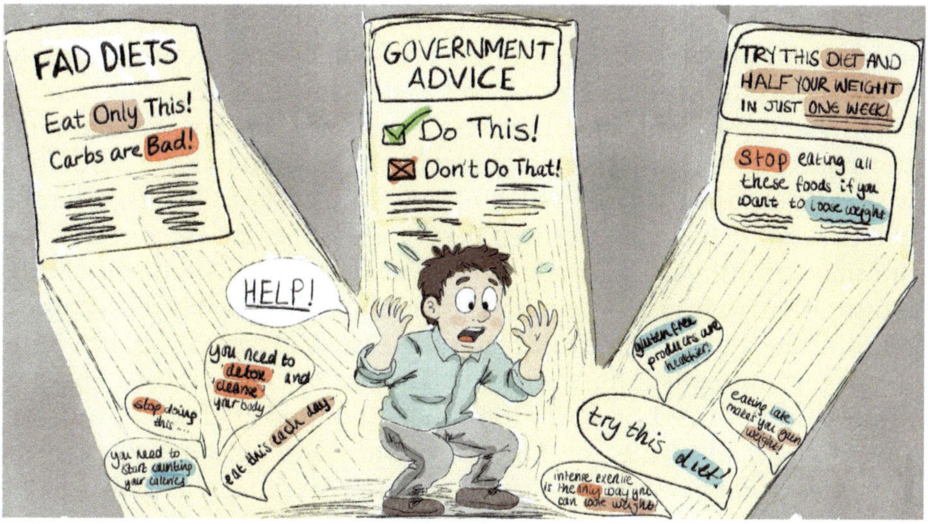

Figure 11.2: Action anxiety.

It Is Time to Take a Chill Pill

Faced with all the distractions and discombobulations of our modern-day food environment and culture, what can we do? The first thing is we need to take a 'chill pill'. Everyone needs to calm down a bit. In Chapter 2, I discussed the role of the hypothalamus in the control of our appetite and metabolism. Our appetite for food has evolved over millions of years, and just like our thirst mechanism tells our brain when we need to drink more water, so too our appetite tells us when we need to eat. As I outlined in Chapter 9, we need to learn to listen to our appetite more and respond to its needs. Of course, I am not suggesting that this is the only solution, nor am I suggesting that our appetite centre is infallible in its signals to us. That said, it would be helpful for us to listen more to our appetitive signals.

One key solution to our current diet confusion is to rid ourselves of our obsession with calories. I appreciate this is easier said than done given the prominence of calories in our modern-day culture. As intimated earlier though, the calorie can be a distraction to adopting a healthy diet. Instead, we should focus on the nutritional content of our food. A basic principle of a healthy diet is its balance and repletion with our daily nutritional requirements. Any fad diet, which encourages you to cut out a particular macronutrient like fat or sugar, is not a healthy option, despite any false promises or claims to the contrary. A healthy diet contains a balance of all essential nutrients. Therefore, any diet deficient in a particular nutrient, by definition, is not healthy. The nutritional content of our diet includes macronutrients like fat, carbohydrate (sugar), protein and fibre (that we met in Chapter 8).

Fat has a bad name and is usually thought of as unhealthy. This is unfortunate as there are healthy forms of fat (such as monounsaturated and polyunsaturated fats from olives and oily fish, respectively) that are healthy options in our diet. Likewise, carbohydrates are a fundamental component of fibre that we obtain from plant-based foods. Therefore, if we eat a plant-based diet (which is favourable for our health), then we will inevitably be ingesting carbohydrates (and calories), but this does not make it unhealthy. In addition to macronutrients, our nutritional requirements also include micronutrients. These are all the vitamins, minerals and other molecules that are essential for the healthy functioning of our cells. There are thousands of micronutrients, and happily we do not need to worry too much about each of them, provided we adopt a healthy diet, and there is no medical reason for deficiency. We obtain these thousands of micronutrients from the plants in our diet, and this is one of the reasons why adopting a plant-based diet is so important. So-called 'superfoods' like broccoli contain an abundance of these essential micronutrients, which is what makes them super. Unfortunately, ultra-processed foods (UPFs) are often deficient in these essential micronutrients, which is one of the multiple reasons they are unhealthy.

At this stage, it is important to point out that there are medical conditions, for example, coeliac disease, rare inborn errors of metabolism or food intolerances and allergies in which there is a requirement for individualised dietary advice. Such specific dietary needs and requirements are extremely important and indeed may be life critical. In such scenarios, of course, it is important that appropriately trained doctors, healthcare professionals, dieticians and medical specialists provide individualised dietary advice and follow-up. It is beyond the scope of this chapter to include specific details about such special medical dietary requirements. Beyond medical concerns, and as outlined at the start of this chapter, we all have our own food preferences that are unique to each of us. Satisfying these food preferences is important for our enjoyment of food.

In this chapter, I keep mentioning 'healthy diet'. But what is meant by a healthy diet? You will have guessed by now, and from the title of this chapter, that there is no single answer to this question. In an ideal world, we would all receive individualised dietary advice and guidance based on our unique nutritional needs that are bespoke to each of us. Realistically though, this is unlikely to happen any time soon (although with the rise of artificial intelligence, who knows what may happen). This realisation provides us with a profound insight into the nature of a healthy diet: it cannot be too prescriptive. A healthy diet needs to take account of our own food preferences to ensure that we enjoy our food: a suggested diet that we do not enjoy, however healthy it may be, will backfire and will not provide a long-term solution. Despite these caveats, it is possible to provide generic advice about healthy diets that we can all strive for. As I keep mentioning, plant-based food is important, as it contains an abundance of fibre and all the micronutrients that we need. Plant-based foods also keep our gut microbiota healthy. Rather than just sticking to one plant, we should eat a variety of plants, indeed the greater the variety the better. A second principle of a healthy diet is to restrict our intake of UPFs. We should cook our food from its raw ingredients where possible, rather than buying pre-prepared and processed foods. Healthy lean meats and poultry, oily fish and dairy products are also healthy. We should try to restrict our intake of sugar and saturated fats, but this aim should be addressed largely through limitation of our intake of UPFs. And that is it! The principles of a healthy diet are simple. I appreciate that there are challenges to the widespread adoption of a healthy diet, and I address these in the last chapter. One of the key messages of this chapter is that apart from the medical exceptions mentioned above, we need to be less prescriptive in our approach to diet. It is not the case that we all need to eat the same foods to have a healthy diet nor can never indulge in a particular food craving that may be unhealthy for us, provided we do not make a habit of it. There are so many foods available to us, and there are multiple examples of a healthy diet. The key to any healthy diet is that it is well balanced nutritionally and that it provides us with all the essential nutrients that we need. This should be a key focus, rather than having distractions and discombobulations by the caloric content of our food or by the latest fad diet. Finally, if we had to choose just one diet, one that has an abundance of scientific supportive evidence and which combines all of the healthy components outlined here, it would be the Mediterranean diet (1).

It Ain't Just the Food, It's the Way That You Eat It

So much for the food content of our diet. However, the concept of diet goes way beyond the nutritional and caloric content of our food. Our eating-related behaviours are also important, and their optimisation should form an essential part of any healthy lifestyle programme. Within the obesity service that I lead, I led the innovation, development and implementation of a mindfulness-based approach to healthy eating. Such an innovative approach to diet and lifestyle forms a key component of the dietary advice that we, as an obesity team, offer our patients. Mindfulness is a way of being, with a focus on one's own internal and immediate external environment in the present moment. Mindfulness means being more aware and attuned to one's environmental signals (and this also includes signals from the body, and is a form of active listening that I discussed in Chapter 9). In the context of eating, mindfulness refers to being aware of every mouthful, to avoid unhealthy snacking, to eat with other people where possible and to avoid mindless forms of eating, where our attention is on something else (such as our favourite soap opera on the TV). We can teach others and ourselves mindfulness. In our obesity service, we showed that mindful eating has multiple benefits that include weight loss, improvements in healthy eating-related behaviours, improvements in self-esteem and confidence in self-management of body weight and even improved compliance with clinic attendances, and engagement with the healthy lifestyles recommended by healthcare professionals (2, 3). In addition to mindfulness, other aspects of our eating behaviours are relevant to our metabolic health. I once coordinated a metabolic study for the BBC on the speed of eating food, and subsequently published research that suggested some metabolic benefits of eating food more slowly in obese women (4). Other studies suggest an association between eating quickly and excessive body weight (5). We should slow down our eating, adopt mindfulness techniques, eat with other people where possible, enjoy our food and avoid eating unhealthy snacks between our main meals.

When in Rome

One of the constraints on the food that we eat is its local availability to us. We can relate to the glorious food available to us when we visit some Mediterranean countries. Fresh tomatoes are super-sized and taste delicious and other fruit and vegetables have become nutritionally supercharged by the Mediterranean sun. We can relate to the wonderful taste of pizza when eaten in Rome or the taste of authentic curry eaten in India. Such incredible food experiences are difficult to replicate when at home. There are good reasons for this that include logistics of transport of key fresh ingredients. As suggested earlier, it is healthy to eat a variety of fresh ingredients. 'When in Rome, eat like the Romans do'. This will not only be a cultural and gustatory experience but will also be a treat for our gut microbiota. All told, it will be a healthy and joyous experience (*fig 11.3*). (There are, of course, the usual precautions to take when travelling, to avoid diarrhoea and food poisoning, which are not such happy experiences!)

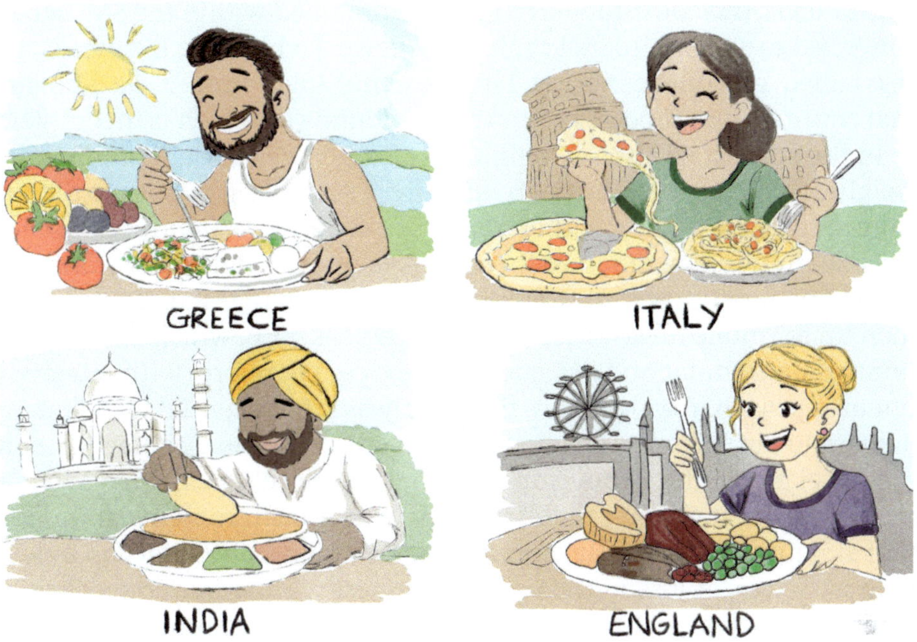

Figure 11.3: When in Rome.

Healthy Diet Versus 'Negative Energy Balance' (NEB)

In Chapter 4, I discussed the importance of SM for metabolic health and the vulnerability of the SM to diminution. In Chapter 10, I discussed the GLP-1 injections ('skinny jabs') and outlined one of the key problems of these therapies regarding their detrimental effect on SM mass and the negative implications this has for our metabolic health. At this point in the chapter, we need to return to this recurrent theme. The key concept that we need to keep in mind throughout these discussions is that the body needs sufficient nutrients each day to keep itself healthy. This includes sufficient energy (the chemical energy that we derive from our food) to drive all the processes within our cells. If this energy threshold is not reached, in other words if the body does not derive its energy requirements from the food that we eat, the body then needs to find an alternate fuel source to power its cells. One option is the fuel contained within our fat cells, and this is one reason why we lose weight when we restrict our caloric intake, due to a reduction in our fat stores. Unfortunately, when our caloric intake is insufficient for our needs, the body also draws on some of its energy requirements from the SM (remember that amino acids, the constituents of protein contained within the SM, can be converted to glucose [to fuel cellular processes] within the liver via a process called 'gluconeogenesis'). There are multiple complex mechanisms that control these processes, our understanding of which is incomplete.

In the context of obesity, weight loss is often desirable. Traditionally, weight loss is achieved through instilling a NEB. This applies to dietary caloric restriction, GLP-1 therapies ('skinny jabs', which reduce appetite and therefore result in reduced caloric intake) and bariatric surgery (in which appetite is also suppressed through changes to the timing of incretin hormone release). In each case, there is NEB, which as explained impacts on both fat and SM energy reserves. Therefore, with our traditional approach to weight loss, there is always the potential for collateral damage to our SM mass and function. As I discussed in Chapter 10, there are novel molecules in development that are more specific for reducing fat mass, whilst sparing the SM, and this approach remains an important aim for obesity management. With that said, a NEB diet can indeed help with weight loss in the context of obesity. However, it needs to be combined with a healthy lifestyle, and ideally with appropriate dietetic support (to ensure a nutritionally replete diet). Furthermore, as I outlined in Chapter 2, we need to be aware of the biological changes to the regulation of appetite and metabolism when we lose weight, and be prepared for weight regain following initial weight loss. Restricting intake of carbohydrates (particularly from UPFs) is a common dietary strategy for losing weight in obesity (6). However, we should understand that the 'low-carbohydrate diet' has its limitations as a long-term dietary strategy.

The reality is that a NEB-based approach to weight loss is far from ideal. We employ it in our traditional approach to the management of obesity, as it is the best option we have currently to help with effective weight loss. This will change in the future, as outlined. Importantly, a NEB-based diet is not the same as a healthy diet. A healthy diet, by definition, contains all the essential nutrients and energy that we need for normal cellular function. A healthy diet is a sustainable option for all of us.

Whose Diet Is It Anyway?

You are the master of your own ship. Your diet is unique to you, and to you alone (well maybe you and your gut microbiota). Listen to your own body and adopt a mindful approach to eating and living. On life's merry journey, in our modern-day world, there will be people who will try to persuade you one way or another along the way. Listen to the true experts and choose a diet that is right and healthy for you. If you have an aversion to roast potatoes, as I used to as a child, then avoid them. Choose foods that you enjoy, but make healthy food choices

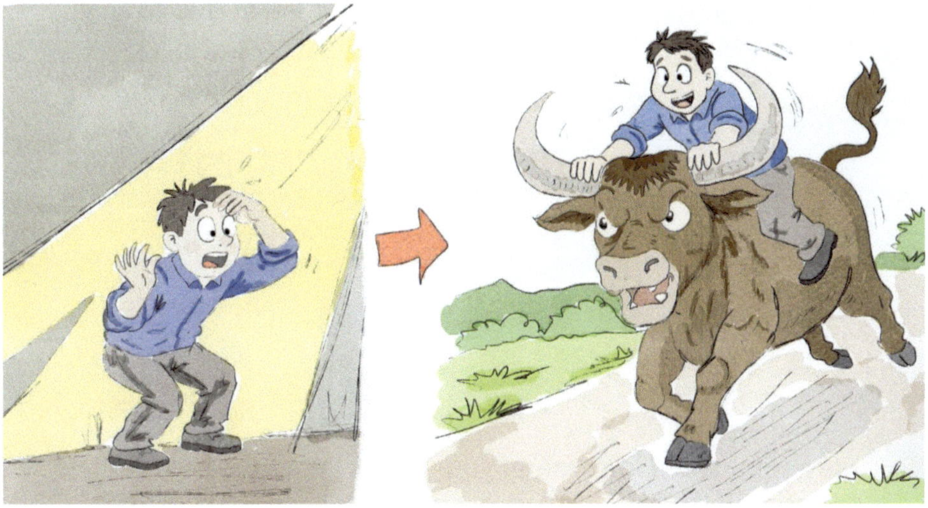

Figure 11.4: Take the bull by the horns.

at the same time. Make time for cooking and experiment with new fresh ingredients. Make eating times a social activity, as a highlight of your day. And when it comes to your food and diet, let us get out of the glare of the startling headlights, and instead take the bull by the horns and go for it (*fig 11.4*).

References

1. Barber TM, Kabisch S, Pfeiffer AFH, Weickert MO. The effects of the mediterranean diet on health and gut microbiota. Nutrients. 2023;15(9):2150.
2. Hanson P, Shuttlewood E, Halder L, Shah N, Lam FT, Menon V, et al. Application of mindfulness in a tier 3 obesity service improves eating behavior and facilitates successful weight loss. J Clin Endocrinol Metab. 2019;104(3):793–800.
3. Hanson P, Lange M, Oduro-Donkor D, Shuttlewood E, Weickert MO, Randeva HS, et al. The role of mindfulness training in sustaining weight reduction: retrospective cohort analysis. BJPsych Open. 2022;8(6):e198.
4. Reddy NL, Peng C, Carreira MC, Halder L, Hattersley J, Piya MK, et al. Enhanced thermic effect of food, postprandial NEFA suppression and raised adiponectin in obese women who eat slowly. Clin Endocrinol (Oxf). 2015;82(6):831–7.
5. Ohkuma T, Hirakawa Y, Nakamura U, Kiyohara Y, Kitazono T, Ninomiya T. Association between eating rate and obesity: a systematic review and meta-analysis. Int J Obes (Lond). 2015;39(11):1589–96.
6. Barber TM, Hanson P, Kabisch S, Pfeiffer AFH, Weickert MO. The low-carbohydrate diet: short-term metabolic efficacy versus longer-term limitations. Nutrients. 2021;13(4):1187.

12 Our Future Transition from Obesogenic to Leptogenic Environment

Take a minute to look around you. This is your own personal physical environment. Note how much of it has been man-made and how much is natural. Note whether there are other people who also occupy your physical environment or whether you are alone. Take note of what sounds you can hear: in my experience, there are always sounds in our environment, whether from the hum of a distant car, the boiler, the washing machine, a dog barking or just the noise of the wind in the trees. There is always something. Then turn your attention to whether there is any food or drink in your immediate environment, the nearest food outlet and the kinds of food available to you (possibly from a mobile electronic device). Now think about the non-physical aspects of your environment, the shared norms, values, beliefs and attitudes within society which we can't point to, but which are just as real to us as this physical book or electronic reading device.

Our environment is everything and everywhere in the current moment and as such is important for our discussion. Our environment has multiple facets. Most obviously, there is the physical environment that surrounds us, in which we conduct our daily lives. Then there is the food environment, which, as its name suggests, relates to the food that is both available and affordable to us. Both physical and food environments vary across multiple criteria, of course, but there are also commonalities. Our cultural environment is perhaps less obvious to us, as it is difficult to step outside of the box and view our society from another vantage point, but we know from history that there have been radical changes to our culture over the centuries in all kinds of ways. We could also imagine an internal environment within our gut, occupied by the gut microbiota, which I discussed in Chapter 5.

In Chapter 1, I discussed our genetic predisposition to obesity, how we all sit on a normal distribution of BMI within our population and how this position is influenced primarily through our genetics. I also mentioned that our genes have not changed in tens of thousands of years, that the rightward shift of the normal distribution for BMI within our population over the last 50-years is usually attributed to our obesogenic environment and more specifically the changes in our environment that have occurred over this time. In this chapter, I discuss what we mean by our modern-day 'obesogenic environment'. I will illustrate this through three aspects of our environment: physical, food and cultural. I will argue that we are all genetic misfits in our modern-day environments and that, to properly address global obesity, we need a redesign of our future environment, to complement our genetics. From the outset, I am not suggesting that we should recreate future environments as mock-ups of the African savanna, but you will see that there is much that we could change if we want to. I use the term 'leptogenic' here to refer to this future imagined environment. As we heard in earlier chapters, leptin is a key hormone released from fat tissue that helps to dampen our appetite and enhance our energy expenditure naturally (that works more efficiently at a healthy body weight), and it is used in this context to denote a future environment that promotes leanness and helps to prevent the onset of obesity. Put simply, a leptogenic environment is one that would enable and facilitate a leftward shift of the normal distribution of BMI within our population. For all their benefits and efficacy at promoting weight loss as outlined in Chapter 10, the GLP-1 injections ('skinny jabs') are only a 'sticking plaster' that mitigate against the weight-gaining propensity of our modern-day maladaptive obesogenic environment. Although these therapies may form part of the solution to global obesity, I believe a much better solution lies within effective and sustainable environmental reform and redesign (1).

Our Obesogenic Environment

Physical

In the context of an obesogenic environment, our physical surroundings are usually included because of their impact on our levels of physical activity and therefore daily energy expenditure (or metabolism): the number of kcals burnt (including within our skeletal muscles [SMs] each day). Over the last few decades, it is incontrovertible that technology has advanced considerably. In many cases, we have innovated such technological advancements to improve our lives, to reduce the need for hard physical exertion and to free up our time for other activities. Notable examples would include the washing machine. I remember as a boy, my grandma had a mangle in the backyard that she would use to wring out the washing after she had handwashed it in the sink. This must have been hard work and time-consuming for her. Nowadays, most of us have washing machines that do all the hard work for us. Transport is another notable example. Driving a car (especially an automatic) doesn't require much physical effort, compared with walking to our destination.

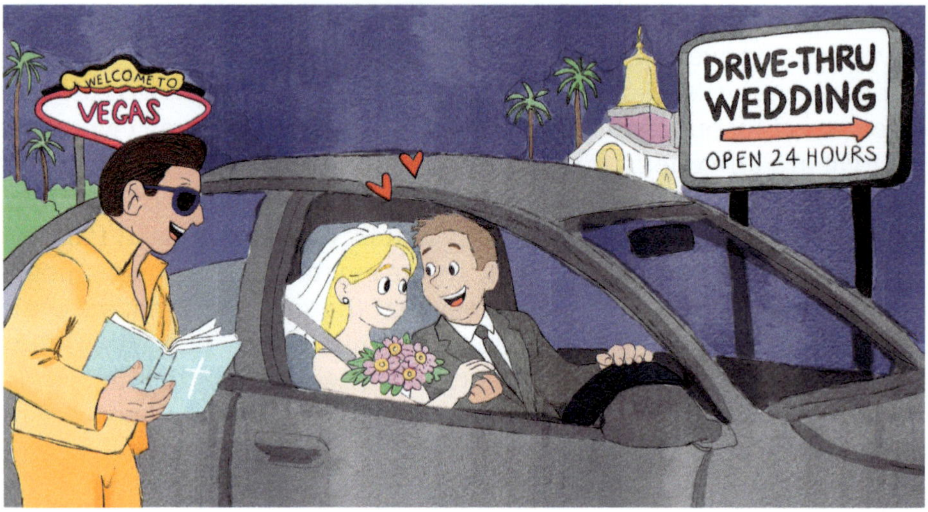

Figure 12.1: Getting married with minimal energy expenditure.

Farming is yet another example: I can't imagine how much effort farmers of the past must have exerted to plough fields with horses, compared with the modern-day equivalent of sitting in a tractor (or even using fully automated machines). When we enter a building, there are often lifts (or elevators if you are reading this in the United States) and escalators or travelators in airports. These technologies are all designed to reduce the amount of physical effort required for us to navigate and move physically through our environments and, of course, to accommodate those of us with physical disablement, an important consideration. Nowadays, we don't even need to leave our car if we want to buy something (often unhealthy!) to eat from a 'drive-through', and in the case of Las Vegas, even to get married (*fig 12.1*).

Beyond technology, we need to consider our built environment and town planning. How much of the human-built environment is designed to optimise healthy forms of transport like walking and cycling, for example? On this point, there may be variations according to where you live, with certain European countries like the Netherlands, for example, having an excellent designed infrastructure for cyclists. We should all learn from the Dutch! Other countries place less emphasis on walking and cycling and instead design towns and cities for the car, in which being a pedestrian can feel alienating. Our towns and cities vary according to the amount of green and open spaces provided for residents to visit on foot and perhaps to engage in physical and social activities. Many spa towns excel at this, and there has been a recent move towards the 'garden town', which in my view is an excellent concept. It can be seen from this discussion that it is not all bad news! In fact, there have been some positive changes to our physical environment in recent years. Furthermore, many of the changes to our physical environment have become manifest gradually since industrialization. I do not believe that changes to our physical environment over the last 50-years caused the global obesity problem, as many of these changes were already in place by the 1970s (although I accept that in some parts of the world this may not have been the case). It is often said that we are more sedentary now than we were 50-years ago and that this sedentariness has contributed towards global obesity. I don't really buy this argument, and I am not aware of any convincing evidence to back up this claim. It may well be that the jobs that we do have become more sedentary, with the rise of computers and technology to replace much traditional physical work, but I don't think we are necessarily more sedentary in our leisure pursuits. In fact, if anything perhaps, we are more physically active. When I was growing up in the 1970s, seeing a jogger on the pavement was an oddity, and gym culture didn't really exist. Now, it is commonplace to see a jogger on the pavement, and gym culture (along with 'health tracking' devices) is big business (2). (I use the example of gyms here as they form part of our physical environment, but gyms have also become part of our modern-day culture).

One other consideration of our modern-day obesogenic environment relates to the ambient temperatures of our living environment. Incredibly, in the 1970s, most homes in the United Kingdom did not have central heating, and average indoor temperatures within homes in the winter were down at a chilly 12°C (brrrrr!). Over a period of just a few decades, the average temperature within UK homes rose by >5°C, due to the rise of central heating (3). You may be wondering why I have chosen to include home temperatures in this discussion of the physical obesogenic environment. The reason is that our daily energy expenditure (metabolic rate, or how many kcals we burn off each day) is influenced by the ambient temperature of our immediate environment. Put simply, we burn off more kcals when our living ambient temperature is cold compared to 'thermoneutrality' (comfortable living temperature). The reason is that we need to burn off more kcals when it is cold to maintain our body temperature (just like your boiler at home needs to work harder and burn more fuel to keep the temperature of your home regulated in the winter when it is cold outside). Although the difference in daily energy expenditure is only around 50 kcals when comparing home environments that differ by 3–5°C on average, over time that may add up. Although we lack convincing evidence, it is possible that warmer indoor living environments may have contributed towards progressive weight gain over the last 50-years, due to a reduction in overall energy expenditure. However, this effect is unlikely to be appreciable.

Food

Of all the facets of our modern-day obesogenic environment, food is often considered the most important. I would agree with this. It is incontrovertible that there were radical changes to our food environment during the late 1970s and 1980s. Of all the contenders for causing the global obesity problem, we would have to place changes to our food environment as number one. When considering these changes to our food environment, it is important to remember that there are multiple components that changed concurrently. Broadly, these can be considered as food composition, availability and affordability.

Our food composition changed radically in the late 1970s and 1980s. In a nutshell, this era saw the widespread introduction and promotion of ultra-processed foods (UPFs), driven by financialisation of food corporations (4). Other key drivers for UPFs included more economical food production, ease of transport and greater shelf life, which were needed due to the rise of the supermarket, rather than its predecessor, the local greengrocery store in which you could (and still can in some locations) buy fresh produce. One problem with fresh food is that it does not keep fresh for long periods, and its shelf life is limited. UPFs overcome this problem. Another driver for UPFs was the widespread belief in the health benefits of low-fat foods that lasted for many decades, and only in recent times has our mindset shifted towards low (or no) sugar food and drinks. In the 1980s, low-fat foods were all the rage. One problem with low-fat foods is that they often require the addition of sugar to make them palatable. Excessive dietary sugar is converted to fat in the liver and therefore contributes towards weight gain. UPFs are typically packed full of sugar. A further problem with UPFs is that they are typically impoverished of any dietary fibre. I discussed the widespread health benefits of dietary fibre in Chapter 8. One of the reasons we are deficient in fibre in our Western diets is because of the widespread ingestion of UPFs. It can be concluded that despite their popularity, UPFs contribute towards weight gain and are often depleted of essential micro- and macronutrients like fibre. We should all limit our ingestion of UPFs.

Food outlets are everywhere, and food availability is widespread. The rise of supermarkets in the 1970s and 1980s meant that shopping for food became convenient. For the first time, you could buy all your weekly shopping (and much else besides) from one shop under one roof, without venturing into multiple shops on the high street and dodging traffic and getting wet in the process. The rise in car ownership made this even more convenient by driving to the supermarket, parking in custom-built car parks and using a trolley to transport your weekly shop directly into your car boot before driving home. These innovations are often taken for granted by us now, but they became properly established at the dawn of the global obesity problem, and they form an important part of our modern-day food environment. To complement supermarkets, the 1970s and 1980s also bore witness to the rise of 'fast-food' outlets, which started popping up all over the place. Although some progress has been made in recent times regarding the healthy food options of at least some fast-food outlets, back in the 1980s, these options were almost all unhealthy. But like supermarkets, they were convenient and increased the ready availability to us of unhealthy food. In our modern-day era of the Information Revolution, food is even more available and accessible to us 24/7, and we can even have it delivered to our homes at the click of a button.

Food also became more affordable to us in the late 1970s and 1980s. Then as now, UPFs were a relatively cheap food option and cheaper than buying healthy raw ingredients. There are multiple drivers for this price disparity, but mass production of UPFs and improved ease of transportation and shelf life are contributors. In many cases (except perhaps at a motorway service station, where everything seems to be relatively expensive), fast food was and continues to be a relatively cheap food option. One of the tragedies of our modern-day food environment is that unhealthy food (often UPFs) tends to be cheaper than healthy food options. In many cases, the poorer members of society can only afford to buy unhealthy foods. It is no coincidence that obesity rates are higher in those from lower socioeconomic groups. If all you can afford is unhealthy UPFs, then how can you possibly hope to adopt a healthy diet and maintain a healthy body weight?

We can think of our modern-day obesogenic food environment as having stemmed from a triple whammy of a profusion of manufactured unhealthy UPFs, being widely and super-conveniently available to and accessible by the populace, at affordable prices. If you had to sit down and design a dreadful prospect for the food environment of humanity, beyond creating a famine, I don't think you could do much worse. How could we have got this so wrong? And why didn't anyone intervene? It gets worse, as we know that some food companies play on the addictiveness of their food products, in an attempt for us, the consumer, to keep buying their product (5). How unethical! Designing foods for the purpose of their addictiveness just to drive profits is, in my view, an evil act. And yet, it seems that some food companies have been allowed to do this, and it is perfectly legal. To me, this seems like a monumental legal loophole, and an elephant in the room when it comes to contributors to the global obesity problem through our food environment. To quote Shakespeare (*The Tempest*), when it comes to our modern-day food environment, it seems that 'Hell is empty, and all the devils are here' (*fig 12.2*).

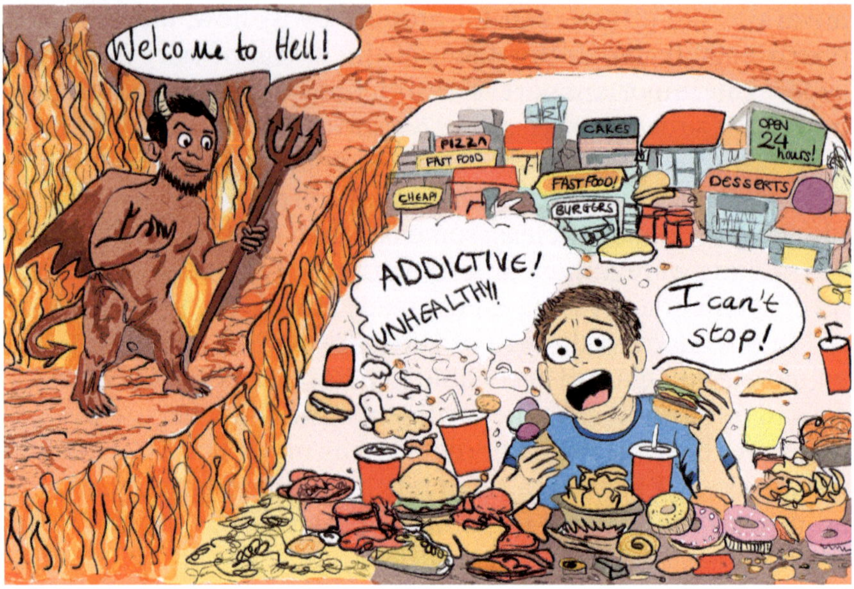

Figure 12.2: A food environment from hell.

Cultural

Compared with our physical and food environments, our cultural environment is more nebulous and difficult to define. Essentially, culture relates to the shared norms, beliefs and values within society. There are many facets of our obesogenic culture, and here I only include a few examples. To complement the changes in our food environment, we also experienced a change in our food culture, with more of us shopping from supermarkets and eating UPFs, for example. This became the norm. It could be said that the widespread belief in the healthiness of low-fat foods formed part of the culture of the 1970s and 1980s, and this cultural belief conspired with the changes in our food environment outlined above to contribute towards weight gain. Likewise, our culture seemed to turn a blind eye to the health hazards of added sugar to our food for many decades, and it only seems to be in recent times, with the introduction of the 'sugar tax' and the option of 'zero-sugar' drinks, for example, that this mindset has started to change. In Chapter 6, I discussed the importance of sleep for our health and for the healthy regulation of our appetite and metabolism. This message of sleep sufficiency as a pillar of healthy lifestyle seems to be missing from our culture. When I was growing up, lifestyle messages that I was taught at school revolved around diet and exercise, and this continues to be the case. Sleep seems to have been ignored and does not seem to be taken as seriously as it should be. Some businesses have undervalued the importance of sleep sufficiency amongst their employees and miscalculated the detrimental impact of sleep deprivation on work productivity and health and well-being, despite an abundance of evidence to support such a link. More recently though, businesses seem to increasingly value sleep sufficiency in their employees.

A Model for a Future Leptogenic Environment

We need to be realistic when we imagine how to optimise our future physical environment. I am not going to suggest that we redesign cars for drivers to be like those driven by Fred Flintstone, powered simply by our legs! Furthermore, we need to be realistic about the scope for a redesigned physical environment. However, it would be helpful for the town planners and architects of the future to have a deep awareness and insight into the physical environment for which we are genetically adapted, and how radically different this is from the one that we inhabit currently in our modern-day world. Whilst our future environment should cater for those with physical disablements, including lifts and escalators and the like, there should also be greater options for able-bodied people to use stairs, for example. Future towns should be designed in a way that promotes healthy forms of transport, including infrastructure for pedestrians and cyclists that are ideally separate from roads, and therefore safer and more efficient to use. These simple measures would help enormously to improve the health and well-being of the populace. There will still be a need and demand for motorised transport. (In the future, our transportation system will likely stem from electrically powered driverless vehicles, with each vehicle communicating with key transport infrastructure and with all other vehicles on the road [similar to our computers and electronic devices being connected with all others through the internet]). Proper infrastructure to enable healthy forms of transport would certainly encourage many of us to utilise these options (including those who are put off by the design of our modern-day urban transport environment, with its typical emphasis on motorised vehicles). In addition to healthy transport infrastructure, our future physical environment should also place an emphasis on greenery rather than concrete jungle. Having plants and trees in one's immediate environment helps with mental health and overall well-being (6). Furthermore, we should encourage people to use healthy forms of transport through making this an enjoyable experience, with surrounding natural environments that are well lit and free from pollution. Having green open spaces with dedicated areas to sit or engage in physical activities like bowls, table tennis or outdoor exercise machines, for example, would encourage people to venture outside of their homes, and would help to facilitate positive social interaction between residents, with an added benefit of helping to address loneliness. Whilst switching from washing machines to mangles is unlikely to be a popular idea, and neither would we want to reverse the technological innovations of the last century, we could still make some other modifications to our home and work environments to improve our metabolism. Having standing desks or dedicated areas within offices to encourage and facilitate engagement of employees in physical activities during break times is one option.

How can we create a redesigned future food environment? There is so much that could be done. The composition of our food should be improved, to provide us with the necessary macro- and micronutrients that our body needs (through added fibre, for example). Future UPFs need to be produced in this way, and food companies should be legally obliged to make this necessary change. In short, UPFs need to be manufactured in a way that promotes improved healthiness rather than merely driving profits. Food companies should be banned from purposely developing UPFs that are addictive to us and should behave more responsibly. However, we shouldn't point the finger entirely at food companies. Governments have just as important a role to play through new legislation and regulations. One irony here is that the drugs that are available to us are under immense scrutiny and regulation, but when it comes to our food, this is simply not the case. And yet, our diet underlies the global obesity problem and much modern-day chronic ill health. The sooner we take our diet seriously, the better. Beyond governments, we all have an important role to play. As consumers, food companies rely upon us for their survival. We can all vote with our mouths and choose healthier food options within our means. We all have the capacity to lobby our MPs and demand improvements to the regulation of our food.

When it comes to food availability, like the idea of switching our washing machines back to mangles, it seems unrealistic, unfeasible and probably undesirable to restrict our food availability. I don't think this idea would win many votes for any political party. However, what I think could work and what should form an important component of the future food environment is increased availability of *healthy* food options. As alluded to earlier, there are some recent examples of this trend. However, the food available to us is still predominantly unhealthy. Walk down any high street in the Western world or visit any fair or market, and this will be obvious to any observer. It could be said that we live in a food desert when it comes to healthy food options. This is understandable: the fact remains that many of us enjoy and derive pleasure from eating unhealthy food. This needs to be balanced though with having healthy food options: including plant-based food that is cooked from its raw ingredients, with olive oil, and avoidance of saturated and trans-fatty acids. Many of us would prefer these healthy food options that nourish our gut, body and

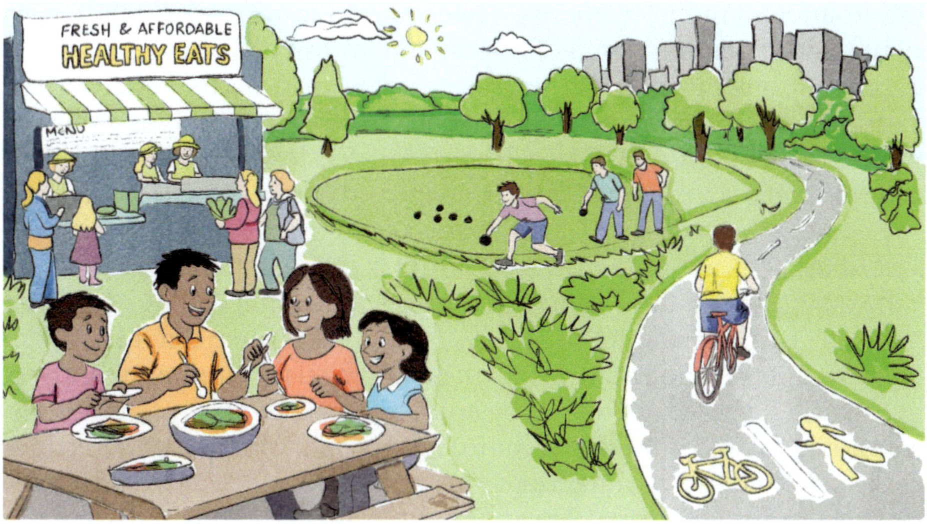

Figure 12.3: A redesigned leptogenic environment.

mind. These options should not just be restricted to food outlets but also apply to our food choices within supermarkets. Rather than restricting healthy food options to one corner of the supermarket with an abundance of unhealthy UPF options that seem to typify many supermarkets, in the future, we should ensure that healthy food options are predominant within our supermarkets. Furthermore, governments should ensure that these healthy food options are affordable to all members of our society. No one should be precluded from having access to affordable healthy food options. For those poorer members of society who may struggle to afford healthy food, governments should intervene to ensure appropriate healthy food subsidies (this could be thought of as the opposite of the sugar tax) to ensure healthy food affordability for all. Such a policy would help to prevent weight gain in the populace, address current inequalities in healthy food affordability and provision and improve overall health and well-being (*fig 12.3*).

It is relatively easy to propose positive changes to our future physical and food environments. Changing our cultural environment is a tougher nut to crack. Why? Because our culture is so complex and nebulous and hidden in plain sight. There is no single aspect to our culture, but rather a complex entity of shared beliefs and values, morphed and formed through innumerable interactions with our peers, teachers, parents and friends and influenced by our personal experiences, upbringing and institutions. Education is important, and the future school environment will play an important role in improving our future cultural environment. Our children need to be taught about diet and sleep, about key life skills including the preparation of healthy meals, to value healthy lifestyles and to understand how obesity develops. These strategies will help to instil a more compassionate outlook and address widespread societal stigmatisation of obesity. Our media can play an important role to avoid stigmatised and depersonalised imagery and language when reporting on obesity-related topics. Healthcare professionals need to lead by example and help the populace to understand obesity and its underlying causes and what we can all do to address this global problem. Whilst the supermarket as an important food outlet is unlikely to change anytime soon, our culture should transition towards a healthier focus on food and eating-related behaviour. Mealtimes should be revered like they are in some Mediterranean countries, with an emphasis on communal eating, an unrushed shared activity to be enjoyed between family and friends. We should all adopt a more mindful approach to our eating behaviour and avoid mindlessness (such as eating unhealthy snacks whilst focusing on some other activity). We should adopt healthy cooking from raw ingredients as the norm. We should value our sleep more and make every effort to improve our sleeping environment and hygiene, to optimise our sleep quality and duration. Finally, influencers on social media should play an important role in any future cultural change to promote a healthy diet and lifestyle and speak and act responsibly in this endeavour.

In the far future, it may become possible for us to change our genes. If not as children or adults, then maybe even *in utero*. Whilst this prospect may seem scary and has huge ethical implications, when it comes to our genetic propensity for weight gain and predisposition to obesity, it is at least possible in principle for our genetics to be modified in a way that could be protective. If and when we reach this stage is anyone's guess, but if we do, it would likely be at least many decades into the future. Although fraught with ethical issues, such innovations in human genetic (and epigenetic) manipulation would provide at least one potential solution to the future global obesity problem. However, even if this innovation were possible, it would not negate the need for positive and sustainable environmental change and the widespread adoption of a healthy lifestyle. Many of the environmental changes suggested here are not just important to optimise our body weight and composition and mitigate against excessive weight gain and the development of obesity, they would also improve our overall health and well-being, regardless of our underlying genetic architecture. A change in our cultural environment would also help to foster population-wide improvement in our understanding of obesity and its causes, an appreciation that none of us are immune from the possibility of weight gain and that our genetic architecture underlies our individual propensities for weight gain and the development of obesity through subtle effects on the settings that control our appetite and metabolism. It is my hope that this book is a stepping stone on a path towards this enlightened status. On this pilgrimage, we can effectively de stigmatise obesity and adopt compassion for those (including ourselves) who gain weight, who live with obesity and its many comorbidities and who live with obesity-related fear and anxiety. As a society, we need courage, fortitude, maturity and insight to make this important cultural change. We all form part of our society, including me and you. We can all make a meaningful impact. The time is now.

Epilogue

Ignorance is part of being human. We are all ignorant. Socrates is considered the wisest person who ever lived, as he openly acknowledged that 'I know that I know nothing'. Such a stance in our modern-day world would likely be met with ridicule and be considered as a weakness. In today's world, it seems that we all need to have an opinion on everything, and it is all about who can shout loudest and disseminate their own opinions to the world, to gain the maximum 'likes', whilst listening less to the opinions of others and not having the courage, fortitude and humility to change or modify one's own opinion based on new evidence or the experiences and insights of others. We should all gain insight from Socrates and accept that we can only ever know a tiny amount of what there is to know, that the more we know, the more we know we don't know and that what we think we know can sometimes (indeed, often) turn out to be incorrect or inaccurate. Furthermore, an important lesson for life is that we can all learn from the experience and insights of others, and we should use this as a mantra. It is in this spirit that I commit this book to the world.

Any working model in science can and should be modified according to novel emergent evidence and insights. Likewise, the contents of this book are true and accurate to the best of my knowledge at the time of its writing. I accept that in years and decades to come, there will likely be new knowledge and insights on obesity that will inevitably change the ways in which we think about it. In just the same way, our knowledge and insights on obesity, its complex pathogenesis and effective management have changed radically even in the last couple of decades.

Although the management of obesity is stratified on a population-wide basis, we are all individuals, and the reality is that we would each benefit from an individualised approach to weight management. However, there are some generic learning points from this book, which are summarised below. Rather than being just another self-help list, I hope that these insights will help you and others you know to adopt a healthy approach to life.

- Obesity, like height, is determined primarily by our genetics. We are all born with a propensity for weight gain which is unique to each of us. Therefore, do not compare your body weight with that of others today, but rather focus on your own body weight that is unique to you, how it has changed over time and the environmental factors that may have influenced this change, and the lifestyle approaches that you can adopt to optimise your own body weight and composition in the future.

- Appetite and metabolism are biological processes controlled by two dimmer switches in the brain and influenced by a myriad of factors, including our underlying genetics. Following loss of body weight, strong biological drivers kick into action to increase your body weight. This is not your own personal failing, but just biology in action. Unfortunately, this does mean that if you lose body weight, it becomes harder and more challenging to maintain your body weight at that new level.
- Do not be too focused on BMI, especially if you are built like Arnie in his prime. Focus more on your body composition, including waist circumference. BMI has all kinds of flaws on an individual level and is not a particularly useful diagnostic tool for obesity.
- Your SM is extremely important for your metabolic health. Optimise, preserve and nurture your SM. Accept that we all lose SM mass as we get older, but we can all adopt lifestyle strategies to mitigate against this process, including regular physical exercise (especially resistance training), combined with optimised protein in the diet. Just like the importance of optimising peak bone mass in our youth (especially in girls and young women) to mitigate against the development of osteoporosis later in life, so too should we appreciate the importance of optimising peak SM mass in our youth to mitigate against the development of obesity and other metabolic problems later in life.
- The gut microbiota is not some alien living within your gut and which eats your food, but rather an essential part of you, and plays a crucial role in optimising your health and well-being and can reduce your risk of developing chronic illness. Develop and nurture your gut microbiota by adopting the healthy lifestyle choices outlined here.
- To sleep, perchance to dream. Sleep more. Take your sleep seriously. Adopt healthy sleep hygiene and ensure that your sleeping environment is optimised for restful sleep. Ensure that your daily routine is conducive to restful sleep and make time in your daily routine to ensure that you get around 7.5 hours of sleep (as an adult) each night, consistently. Stick to a regular sleep-wake cycle.
- Interrupt prolonged sedentariness with regular brief periods of light physical activity. Ensure that you get good amounts of physical activity each day by using your SMs and if you are able,

try to engage in regular physical exercise, the type that brings you in a sweat.
- Eat more plants every day and diversify the types of plants you eat.
- Listen.
- Pharmacotherapy is not *the* solution to the global obesity problem. Rather, pharmacotherapy provides a sticking plaster applied to a wound that has been created by a mismatch between our genetics and our modern-day obesogenic environment. Pharmacotherapy may play an important role in facilitating weight loss in some, but this should not be seen as a commodity, but rather a serious drug therapy that should only be used in the context of appropriate specialist medical assessment and follow-up. Furthermore, as with any drug therapy, there are potential tolerability and safety issues that need to be considered carefully on an individual basis.
- There is a myriad of fad diets out there, many of which have little or no scientific supporting evidence. If you need to choose one, the Mediterranean diet has more supportive evidence for its health benefits than any other. We are all unique in our dietary needs and requirements. Do not get distracted by our obsession with the kcal, but rather choose foods based on their macro- and micronutrient content. Wherever possible, cook from raw ingredients, and limit your intake of UPFs.
- The global obesity problem reflects environmental changes since the early 1970s, specifically to our physical, food and cultural environments. To truly address the global obesity problem will require us to transform our obesogenic environment to a leptogenic environment. Anything else is merely a sticking plaster.

To quote Rudyard Kipling: If you can achieve all of this... 'Yours is the Earth and everything that's in it'.

We are nearly done, but I wanted to finish on a human note. None of us are machines or automatons. To err is human, and as humans, we make mistakes. Furthermore, application of the healthy lifestyles outlined here can be difficult and challenging for all of us, particularly at times of personal stress or following a life event. We need to acknowledge and embrace our human frailties. In this acceptance, let us walk with our modern-day human family in the footsteps of our ancient hominid ancestors, to attain true happiness, fulfilment and inner peace, and in the process make the world a better place for all.

After all, to quote the legendary American golfer, Walter Hagen:

> *'You're only here for a short visit.*
> *Don't hurry, don't worry. And be sure to smell the flowers along the way'. (fig 12.4)*

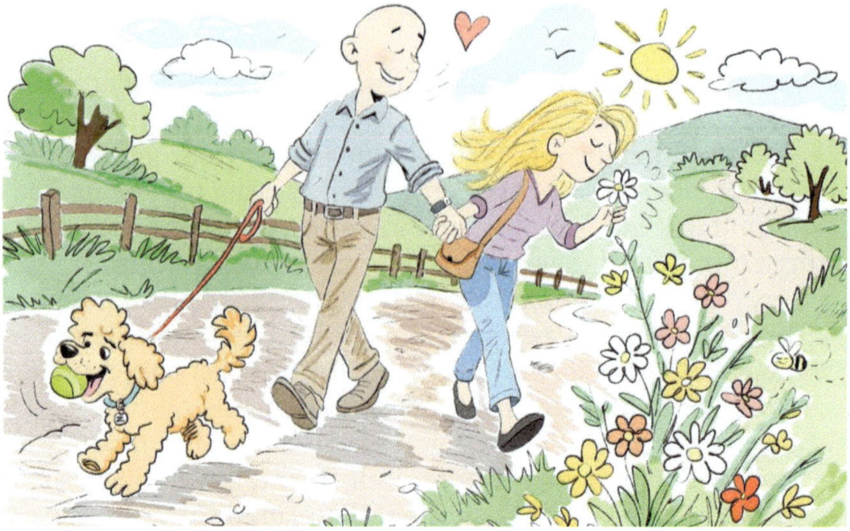

Figure 12.4: Smell the flowers along the way.

References

1. Hanson P, Weickert MO, Barber TM. Obesity: novel and unusual predisposing factors. Ther Adv Endocrinol Metab. 2020;11:2042018820922018.
2. Kristensen DB, Kuruoglu AP, Banke S. Tracking towards care: relational affordances of self-tracking in gym culture. Sociol Health Illn. 2021;43(7):1598–613.
3. Mavrogianni A, Johnson F, Ucci M, Marmot A, Wardle J, Oreszczyn T, et al. Historic variations in winter indoor domestic temperatures and potential implications for body weight gain. Indoor Built Environ. 2013;22(2):360–75.
4. Wood B, Robinson E, Baker P, Paraje G, Mialon M, van Tulleken C, et al. What is the purpose of ultra-processed food? An exploratory analysis of the financialisation of ultra-processed food corporations and implications for public health. Global Health. 2023;19(1):85.
5. LaFata EM, Allison KC, Audrain-McGovern J, Forman EM. Ultra-processed food addiction: a research update. Curr Obes Rep. 2024;13(2):214–23.
6. Wang R, Helbich M, Yao Y, Zhang J, Liu P, Yuan Y, et al. Urban greenery and mental wellbeing in adults: cross-sectional mediation analyses on multiple pathways across different greenery measures. Environ Res. 2019;176:108535.

Index

A

B

F

G

H